MW01489924

TOXIC NEST

The Dirt Behind 'Clean'

By Jenece Mordt M.Ed

© 2025 Jenece Mordt M.Ed. All rights reserved.

No part of this publication may be reproduced, stored in a retrieval system, or transmitted by any means—electronic, mechanical, photocopying, recording, or otherwise—without the prior written permission of the author, except in the case of brief quotations used in reviews or articles.

Printed in the United States of America.
ISBN: 9798280902770
First Edition, 2025

Disclaimer: The information provided in this book is for educational and informational purposes only. It is not intended as medical advice or as a substitute for medical treatment. Always consult with a qualified healthcare provider before making changes to your health, home, or lifestyle practices.

"Every truth passes through three stages: It is ridiculed, it is violently opposed, and finally, it is accepted as self-evident."

—Arthur Schopenhauer

Introduction

We assume our homes are safe.
Clean. Controlled.
Our refuge from the chaos outside.

But what if the very space we rely on for rest and recovery is quietly making us sick?

In *Toxic Nest: The Dirt Behind 'Clean'*, author, Jenece Mordt peels back the sanitized layers of modern domestic life to reveal the invisible chemical exposures that surround us, from "fresh-scented" cleaners to flame-retardant crib mattresses, microplastic-laced pajamas, and greenwashed baby wipes.

This book is not about panic. It's about power.

Drawing from scientific research, ancestral wisdom, and stories from real women, Jenece offers a sobering and empowering journey through the modern home, room by room. She explores how synthetic materials, fragranced products, and industrialized living have disrupted not only our health, but our hormonal balance, mental clarity, maternal instinct, and sense of safety.

And she offers a path forward, not through fear or perfectionism, but through awareness, agency, and practical steps that restore the home as a sacred, life-supporting space.

For mothers, caregivers, healers, and anyone ready to reclaim their environment, *Toxic Nest* is a wake-up call, and a deeply personal call to action.

Because before we can protect the next generation, we have to protect the nest. And to do that, we must be willing to see the truth behind what we've been sold as "clean."

Chapter 1:

The Polluted Nest

We think of home as a refuge.
A nest, safe, warm, and protective.
But in the modern world, that nest has been quietly polluted.

The air inside our homes, once assumed to be cleaner than the outside, is often laced with invisible toxins. Volatile organic compounds (VOCs), mold spores, and synthetic fragrances drift silently through nurseries, bedrooms, and living rooms, polluting our breath without scent, symptom, or sound. According to the EPA, indoor air can be up to five times more polluted than outdoor air. And yet, we trust it implicitly.

We breathe it in while cooking, cleaning, nursing, and sleeping. Our children crawl through it, play in it, nap inside it. But behind the "fresh scent" and sterile shine lies a chemical fog we were never warned about, and that few of us even notice.

Until our bodies do.

A Familiar Story

A few years ago, a woman I chatted with, let's call her Sara, moved into a newly renovated townhouse with her husband and toddler. The place looked perfect: fresh white paint, sleek laminate flooring, recessed lighting, and that faint floral scent of plug-in air fresheners humming softly in every room. It was everything she'd hoped for, a clean, beautiful space to build their next chapter.

But within a week, her toddler developed a dry, relentless cough that wouldn't go away. Her husband started waking up with headaches and burning eyes. Sara, who had always been clear-minded and even-keeled, began to feel like she was unraveling: dizzy spells, constant fatigue, brain fog, and a tight, unsettled feeling in her chest every time she walked through the door.

At first, she blamed the usual suspects, stress, the adjustment period, maybe seasonal allergies. But the pattern didn't lie: the symptoms flared at home and disappeared when they were away. A weekend trip to visit her parents brought relief. A long afternoon at the park felt like medicine. Returning home felt like stepping back into a fog she couldn't name.

Doctors offered no answers. Tests were inconclusive. "Maybe it's anxiety," one suggested. "Maybe you just need to rest more," said another. But Sara knew something deeper was wrong.

Out of desperation, she hired an independent indoor air quality specialist. The results were shocking: dangerously high levels of formaldehyde were off-gassing from the brand-new flooring, cabinetry, and pressed wood furniture. The plug-in air fresheners were adding a steady stream of phthalates and VOCs to the mix. The

very things that made the house look and smell "clean"
were filling the air with toxins.

It wasn't a virus. It wasn't bad parenting.
It wasn't her imagination.
It was the house.

Sara began making changes, removing synthetic
scents, opening windows, running air purifiers, replacing
high-off gassing furniture with low-tox alternatives. And
slowly, the fog lifted. Her son's cough faded. Her
husband's headaches disappeared. And for the first time
in months, she felt like herself again.

This isn't an isolated story. It's not rare.
It's a pattern, one unfolding in homes across the country.
Quiet. Invisible. Unacknowledged.
But devastating just the same.

The VOC Problem

Volatile Organic Compounds—or VOCs—are found
in an astonishing number of household materials. They
off-gas invisibly from paints, varnishes, adhesives, air
fresheners, cosmetics, mattresses, furniture, carpets,
flooring, and cleaning sprays. They are often odorless, or
masked with synthetic fragrance to seem "fresh," but the
air they create is anything but.

Short-term exposure to VOCs is linked to
headaches, dizziness, nausea, fatigue, skin irritation, and

burning eyes or throat. But it's the long-term exposure—daily, chronic, often unrecognized—that's more insidious. VOCs have been associated with hormonal disruption, reproductive issues, nervous system dysfunction, kidney and liver damage, and various forms of cancer (NIH, 2021). Some VOCs, like formaldehyde and benzene, are classified as known human carcinogens.

This is not just an industrial problem. It's a household one.

A 2018 study by the California Air Resources Board revealed that common consumer products—hair sprays, body sprays, deodorants, perfumes, surface cleaners, disinfectant wipes, and air fresheners—collectively emit as much VOC pollution as all cars and trucks in the state. That's not a metaphor. That's measurable atmospheric load.

And inside the tightly sealed boxes we now call homes, those emissions don't dissipate. Modern construction emphasizes airtight insulation for energy efficiency, but at the cost of air exchange. What we save in heating bills, we pay for in stagnant, chemical-laden air that builds up day after day.

In poorly ventilated homes, especially in winter or in newer builds, this creates a low-grade chemical smog, trapped within the walls we trust.

Who It Hurts Most

VOCs don't affect everyone equally. Like all environmental toxins, they hit the most vulnerable first and hardest.

- Children breathe faster than adults and spend more time close to the floor, where VOC concentrations tend to settle due to chemical density and low airflow. Their skin is more permeable. Their detox organs are immature. Their bodies are smaller, meaning dose-to-weight exposure is significantly higher.

- Pregnant women face additional risk, as VOCs can cross the placental barrier, affecting fetal development, hormone signaling, and neurological growth.

- People with asthma, allergies, or autoimmune conditions often experience flares or symptom spikes in response to VOC exposure—even when they can't smell a thing.

There is no "safe level" of formaldehyde for a toddler. There is no "acceptable dose" of benzene in the nursery. Yet many families are unknowingly living in daily contact with these substances—through the very materials and products they were told were necessary to keep a house "clean."

The Mold Factor

While VOCs are synthetic, another equally dangerous invader is biological: mold. Mold doesn't come with a warning label. It doesn't need to be applied or sprayed. It grows silently in the background, feeding on moisture, cellulose, and time.

Mold thrives in dark, damp, stagnant environments: basements, bathrooms, under sinks, inside HVAC systems, behind wallpaper, underneath flooring, and within drywall or cabinetry. The scariest part? You don't need to see it—or even smell it—for it to wreak havoc.

Not all mold is visible. Not all musty smells are obvious. And not all mold is "black mold." Many strains are colorless or hidden behind walls, but still produce mycotoxins—dangerous compounds released into the air that can travel through ventilation systems and settle in household dust.

The Health Toll of Hidden Mold

The symptoms of mold exposure are often vague, chronic, and misdiagnosed. People may go months—or even years—without realizing that the root of their suffering is microbial.

Common symptoms include:

- Chronic fatigue and low energy

- Brain fog, forgetfulness, and poor concentration

- Histamine intolerance and allergic reactions

- Hormonal dysregulation (especially cortisol and thyroid imbalances)

- Respiratory distress, wheezing, and frequent sinus infections

- Anxiety, mood swings, and even depressive symptoms

In people with mold sensitivity, autoimmune conditions, or compromised detox systems, even low-level exposure can be debilitating. Children are particularly vulnerable, as their lungs, immune systems, and brains are still developing.

The Modern Mold Trap

Today's homes are often designed to seal us in, not to let the building breathe. In the name of energy efficiency, newer construction uses materials that trap moisture and limit ventilation: synthetic insulation, vapor barriers, plastic-lined drywall, and sealed windows that barely open. Add in moisture from showers, cooking, laundry, and seasonal humidity, and you have the perfect storm for mold to flourish.

According to the World Health Organization, over 30% of buildings worldwide have some form of indoor dampness or mold contamination (WHO, 2009). In the U.S., that number may be even higher in climates with poor building codes, high rainfall, or widespread use of "fast-build" materials after natural disasters.

And unlike VOCs, mold isn't just a product of consumer choice, it's a systemic construction failure. You didn't "choose" mold. You were never taught to look for it. And most home inspections barely scratch the surface.

The Mold Denial Problem

Most mainstream doctors still don't test for mold-related illness. Many dismiss it entirely. And few building professionals are trained to detect it accurately, especially when it hides behind walls or under floors.

As a result, people suffer in silence. They move from one prescription to the next. They're told it's "all in their head." But deep down, they know something in their environment is off. Their bodies are telling the truth that the system won't name.

The Good News? Mold Can Be Found—and Remediated.

If you suspect mold, trust your gut. Look for:

- Persistent musty smells (especially in closets, bathrooms, or basements)

- Cold spots or water stains on walls or ceilings

- Chronic condensation on windows

- Symptoms that worsen at home and improve when away

If needed, hire an independent mold inspector, not just a basic home inspector. Look for someone certified in ERMI or HERTSMI testing who uses air sampling, moisture meters, and thermal imaging.

And above all, know this: You are not crazy. You are not fragile. You are not alone. You are responding—brilliantly—to something real.

Fragrance as Pollution

One of the most insidious sources of indoor air pollution is also one of the most culturally accepted and even celebrated. Fragrance.

We spray it. We plug it in. We pour it into our laundry and scrub it into our floors. We light candles with names like "Fresh Rain" and "Ocean Breeze," and we associate those scents with cleanliness, comfort, and care.

But fragrance, in the modern world, is not made from flowers and herbs. It is made from chemicals. And many of those chemicals are quietly harming the very people who use them most.

Fragrance formulations are considered proprietary. Under current labeling laws, companies are allowed to list "fragrance" or "parfum" on an ingredient label without disclosing any of the actual substances used. That single word can represent a cocktail of up to 100 or more synthetic chemicals, many of which are known to impact human health.

Common components of fragrance mixtures include:

- Phthalates, used to help scent stick to skin or fabric. These are known endocrine disruptors that interfere with hormone signaling and have been linked to reproductive abnormalities, thyroid dysfunction, and early puberty.

- Formaldehyde, a known carcinogen that may be used as a preservative or byproduct of other ingredients in fragrance blends.

- Synthetic musks, which are persistent in the environment and in human tissue. These compounds bioaccumulate, meaning they build up in fat stores over time and can interfere with estrogen pathways and detoxification processes.

Fragranced products are now a primary source of indoor air contamination, surpassing even some industrial pollutants. When you use a scented laundry detergent or plug-in air freshener, you are not just adding a pleasant aroma. You are releasing a vaporized chemical cloud into your airspace, one that lingers on surfaces, clothing, bedding, and in the air itself long after the product is applied.

For sensitive individuals, the effects can be immediate. Headaches. Nausea. Dizziness. Asthma attacks. For others, the damage is more gradual and invisible. Disrupted sleep. Elevated cortisol. Subtle shifts in mood, digestion, or menstrual cycles. Hormonal noise that adds up quietly over time.

And yet we are taught to see these products as essential. Clean homes are supposed to smell like something—lavender, citrus, pine, vanilla. Unscented spaces are labeled as sterile or neglected. We've been conditioned to fear the absence of fragrance rather than question its presence.

But what we think of as "fresh" is often the scent of petrochemical derivatives, alcohols, solvents, and hormone-disrupting compounds released into our living space and absorbed through our skin, lungs, and bloodstream.

This is not about paranoia. It is about informed consent. It is about knowing what you are breathing and absorbing. It is about recognizing that true cleanliness is scent-neutral, not artificially perfumed. And it is about shifting the narrative from masking odors to actually reducing the toxins that create them in the first place.

To detox the air in your home, removing synthetic fragrance is one of the most powerful steps you can take. It costs nothing to unplug the device. It takes only a moment to switch to a fragrance-free detergent. It may feel uncomfortable at first, because the silence of a scentless space can feel unfamiliar. But over time, that quiet becomes a form of clarity. You begin to smell life again—wood, rain, lemon zest, baby skin, clean air.

And in that clarity, the body begins to settle.

What You Can Do

This chapter isn't about scaring you into silence or shame-it's about inviting you into awareness and action. Here are some first steps you can take to begin reclaiming your indoor air:

- Ventilate often. Open windows, especially during cleaning or cooking.

- Go fragrance-free. Choose unscented or naturally scented (essential oil-based) products.

- Ditch the plug-ins and sprays. They are among the worst offenders.

- Use an air purifier. Look for HEPA filters with activated carbon.

- Check for mold. Trust your senses and investigate any musty areas. If necessary, hire a professional mold inspector-not just a standard home inspector.

- Choose low- or no-VOC materials. Especially when buying new mattresses, furniture, or paint.

Most of all, trust your instincts. If you or your children feel foggy, irritable, allergic, or exhausted at home-your body is speaking. The air around you might be speaking too.

Up next: What's under the sink-and why the cleanest-looking products might be the most harmful.

Chapter 2:

The Clean That Kills

Walk down the cleaning aisle of any store and you'll be hit with a wall of scent so thick it clings to your clothes and follows you home. Citrus, lavender, ocean breeze, chemical imitations of nature, engineered to evoke safety, care, and control. These scents are designed to sell the idea that we're protecting our families.

But behind the bright labels and fresh smells lies a darker truth: many of the most common cleaning products are toxic by design.

The very substances we use to sanitize and defend our homes are filled with compounds that irritate the lungs, disrupt hormones, suppress immune function, and may contribute to chronic disease. The irony is stark. In our efforts to kill germs, we are often poisoning our nests.

The Problem with Cleaners

Most commercial cleaning products are not what they seem. The labels are bright, the scents are cheerful, the promises are confident—"Kills 99.9% of germs," "Tough on grease," "Fresh scent." But behind the branding lies a murky truth: these bottles often contain unlisted, unregulated, and untested chemical compounds that can do more harm than the dirt they're meant to clean.

Most cleaning formulas include a combination of surfactants, solvents, preservatives, pH adjusters, dyes, and synthetic fragrances. These ingredients interact chemically, degrade over time, and off-gas into your home's air and dust, especially in warm, humid conditions like kitchens and bathrooms.

Here's the real problem: you're not told what's in them.

Unlike food or cosmetics, cleaning products are not legally required to list all their ingredients. Read that again, cleaning products are not legally required to list all their ingredients. In the United States, the Consumer Product Safety Act allows companies to withhold ingredient information by citing "trade secrets." So one word—*fragrance*—can legally represent dozens or even hundreds of hidden chemicals. And terms like "green," "natural," and "eco-friendly" are unregulated, making them meaningless when it comes to safety.

That means a bottle labeled "gentle lemon cleaner" might contain:

- Ethanolamines, which can react with other ingredients to form carcinogenic nitrosamines

- Synthetic musks that can build up in fat and breastmilk

- Quaternary ammonium compounds (quats) linked to decreased fertility and thyroid dysfunction

- 1,4-dioxane, a byproduct of the ethoxylation process and a probable human carcinogen according to the

These aren't rare contaminants. They're commonly found in top-selling household brands. Some are even found in products marketed specifically for nurseries and baby care.

What's worse, manufacturers are not required to test how these chemicals interact in combination, or how they accumulate over time in the body.

This is not just a labeling issue. It's a regulatory failure.

The last major piece of U.S. federal legislation regulating household chemicals was passed in 1976. The Toxic Substances Control Act (TSCA) grandfathered in more than 60,000 chemicals already in use, assuming them safe unless proven otherwise. Only a tiny fraction of those have ever been formally tested for long-term health effects.

So when you clean your kitchen with a commercial spray, you're not just wiping up crumbs. You're aerosolizing unlisted chemicals into your breathing space. You're coating your counters with hormone disruptors. You're absorbing solvents through the skin of your hands, and your children's hands, and their mouths, when they eat off that surface.

This is the silent side of "clean."
And most people have no idea it's happening.

A Familiar Story

Renee was a mom of three under five, with a minivan and a perfectly organized pantry. She sprayed countertops multiple times a day, bleached the bathtub weekly, and never ran laundry without scent boosters. She thought she was doing everything right.

But she was exhausted. Her skin was constantly irritated, her youngest developed a persistent cough, and her middle child began reacting to everything—dust, foods, even the couch.

A chance article about cleaning product toxicity sent her down a rabbit hole. Within a week, she swapped her disinfectant wipes for vinegar spray, removed all synthetic scents, and switched to unscented detergent. Two weeks later, the cough disappeared. Her own headaches faded. The house felt calmer, clearer, more alive.

Renee didn't stop cleaning. She started cleaning *differently.*

A Historical Detour: Cleanliness and Control

To understand how we got here—how we ended up scrubbing our homes with hormone disruptors and spraying our nurseries with chemical fog—we need to look at the cultural story that made it normal.

Because the way we clean today didn't come from science. It came from advertising. From industry. From control.

In the late 19th and early 20th centuries, Western societies began to equate cleanliness with morality, modernity, and social status. Public health campaigns linked hygiene with patriotism and civic duty. At the same time, industrial capitalism began producing synthetic soaps and cleaners at scale, making cleanliness not just a virtue, but a commodity.

By the 1920s and 1930s, cleaning products were marketed directly to women as their moral and maternal responsibility. Companies framed domestic mess as a source of shame, and offered chemical solutions in brightly labeled bottles. Advertisements targeted women's fears: of being a bad mother, a bad wife, a failure.

Lysol ran ads suggesting that cleanliness kept a husband's love. Pine-Sol declared that dirty floors meant you didn't care. And "germs" were no longer just microbial threats, they were stand-ins for poverty, failure, and female inadequacy.

By the 1950s, the chemical industry—fueled by World War II technology—flooded the consumer market with new substances. Many were industrial-grade solvents, plasticizers, or synthetic fragrances repurposed for household use. The home became a testing ground for these new tools of domestic control.

The messaging was crystal clear:
A good woman used bleach.
A good mother kept a fresh-smelling home.
A good wife never let her bathroom smell like real life.

And in the process, cleanliness became performance.

It was no longer about removing dirt. It was about removing evidence of living.

A truly clean home didn't just look spotless. It smelled synthetic. It shone. It sparkled. It had no trace of mess, body, or nature. That was the goal, and that goal was sold in every aisle, on every shelf, in every magazine ad aimed at women who just wanted to do right by their families.

What We Lost in the Process

What got erased in this chemical campaign was the truth: real clean isn't sterile. It isn't covered in fake lemon scent. It doesn't need to burn your eyes or trigger your asthma to be effective.

Traditional cleaning methods—vinegar, sun drying, essential oils, baking soda, boiling water, fresh air—were quietly dismissed as old-fashioned, ineffective, or unsanitary. And along with them, ancestral knowledge, maternal intuition, and natural rhythms were pushed to the margins.

This didn't happen by accident.
It happened by design.

Because once cleanliness became industrial, it became profitable. And once it became profitable, it had to be maintained through fear, shame, and aspiration.

And still today, those messages linger. When a mother doesn't use a disinfectant wipe, she's considered careless. When a house smells like nothing, it feels "off." When a floor isn't scrubbed with brand-name chemicals, it feels unfinished.

But all of that was planted.

And we're allowed to uproot it.

How These Chemicals Affect Us

While acute poisonings from cleaning products are relatively rare, long-term, low-dose exposure is a growing focus in environmental health. The body does not always react with a dramatic collapse, it whispers. It shifts subtly. And over time, those whispers become symptoms that no one seems able to explain.

We are not just encountering one chemical at a time. We are layering them—day after day, breath after breath—on our skin, in our lungs, in the rooms where we sleep and raise our children.

The most common impacts include:

- Respiratory issues: Cleaners containing bleach, ammonia, and quats can irritate the lungs, trigger asthma, and exacerbate chronic bronchitis. Children exposed to frequent disinfectant use at home have been shown to have higher rates of wheezing and reduced lung function.

- Endocrine disruption: Many cleaning agents contain substances that mimic or block hormone activity—like phthalates, parabens, and synthetic musks. These disrupt estrogen, testosterone, thyroid hormones, and cortisol balance, leading to menstrual irregularities, low fertility, fatigue, and mood disorders.

- Skin allergies and chemical sensitivities: Preservatives like methylisothiazolinone are known to cause contact dermatitis, eczema, and rashes, especially in children. Over time, repeated exposure can lead to chemical sensitivity syndromes, where the body becomes reactive to even small amounts of toxins.

- Neurological and developmental effects: Exposure to certain solvents and synthetic fragrances is linked to neurotoxicity, brain fog, and attention issues. For children, the effects can be even more profound, impacting neurodevelopment, behavior, and emotional regulation.

One landmark 2018 study published in *The American Journal of Respiratory and Critical Care Medicine* found that women who regularly used chemical cleaning products experienced lung function decline equivalent to smoking a pack of cigarettes a day (Svanes et al., 2018). The damage was not seen in men, underscoring the gendered nature of this exposure, because women, especially mothers, are more often the ones cleaning.

Chronic Exposure Is Not a Coincidence

We tend to think of health events as isolated—headaches, mood changes, skin reactions, or fertility struggles. But our bodies don't work in silos. Every system is interconnected. And toxic exposures, even at low doses, can ripple through the endocrine system, the immune system, and the nervous system in ways that compound over time.

Most products are tested for short-term irritation or accidental ingestion, not for daily inhalation, low-dose absorption, or cumulative impact over decades. And no one is testing how these chemicals interact with one another inside the human body. We are the experiment.

It is no coincidence that so many women report:

- Brain fog

- Worsening PMS or early menopause

- Anxiety and fatigue that defy lab results

- Children with chronic respiratory or behavioral issues

It's not in your head. It's in your household load.

This Is Not About Fear—It's About Awareness

You don't have to be scared to be clear.
You don't have to live in a bubble.
You don't have to throw everything away.

You just need to understand what's actually happening when you spray that surface cleaner.
What's entering the air when you wash with that lemon-scented wipe.
What's settling into your child's skin as they crawl across a just-mopped floor.

And from that awareness, you get to choose something different.
Something that cleans your home without hurting the people inside it.

The COVID Catalyst

When the COVID-19 pandemic began, cleanliness took on a whole new weight. In a matter of weeks, wiping down surfaces became a ritual of survival. Families sanitized groceries. Parents sprayed strollers. Teachers fogged classrooms. Hand sanitizer was stashed in every bag, car, and hallway.

We weren't just cleaning anymore, we were disinfecting compulsively, often without understanding what we were spraying, what it contained, or how it might affect our long-term health.

And the cleaning industry seized the moment.

Sales of disinfectant products surged by over 230% in 2020 alone, and marketing campaigns leaned hard into fear: "Protect your loved ones." "Eliminate invisible threats." "Sanitize everything." But many of these products were not harmless.

Most consumers were using industrial-grade disinfectants, containing quaternary ammonium compounds (quats), chlorine, ethanolamines, and artificial fragrance blends—multiple times per day, often in poorly ventilated spaces.

These chemicals were not tested for safe chronic exposure, especially for children. Nor were they meant to be inhaled daily, layered across multiple surfaces, or used by pregnant women and people with asthma or autoimmune conditions. Yet the public was never warned. In fact, they were praised for over-sanitizing.

The Illusion of Control

Disinfecting became more than a public health measure, it became a psychological coping mechanism. For many people, especially mothers, cleaning became the only form of control they had during a time of deep uncertainty and chaos.

The house became the last frontier. The only thing we could keep "safe."

Mothers, especially, bore the brunt. They were expected to homeschool, work remotely, care for their families, and maintain a sanitized environment. And every brand capitalized on that pressure, offering antibacterial everything in pastel bottles, marketed as self-care, as maternal duty, as love.

But few were asking the deeper questions:

- What are we inhaling every time we spray these products?

- What are we exposing our children to in the name of cleanliness?

- What is happening to our microbiomes, our lungs, and our hormones?

And what if, in trying to kill one threat, we were inviting in another?

What the Science Actually Shows

By mid-2021, it became clear that fomite transmission—the spread of COVID-19 through surfaces—was extremely rare. The virus spread primarily through airborne droplets, not kitchen counters or mail packages. And yet, by then, the damage was done.

We had trained a generation of children to be afraid of touching anything.
We had fogged classrooms with chemicals that irritate lungs and disrupt hormones.
We had layered toxic compounds into our breathing space in the name of protection.

This was not an accident.
It was a failure of public health messaging, corporate ethics, and collective memory.

What We Learned

The pandemic didn't just change how we clean. It exposed how vulnerable we are to chemical manipulation through fear. It showed how quickly companies can flood homes with untested, harmful products when consumers are desperate for safety.

But it also opened the door for new awareness.

Many mothers began reading labels. Many families began asking harder questions.
And many began to realize that real protection isn't about wiping harder. It's about breathing easier.

How Cleaning Culture Targets Mothers

No one is more impacted by cleaning culture than mothers.

We are told—explicitly and implicitly—that a clean home is a moral obligation. That it reflects our character, our competence, and our care for our children.

But what happens when "clean" is actually harmful?

Mothers are disproportionately exposed to cleaning chemicals, and disproportionately blamed when something goes wrong: a sick child, a messy room, a chronic cough.

This chapter isn't about adding guilt. It's about removing it—by giving mothers the information they were never told, and the permission to clean *for health*, not for appearance.

Reclaiming Real Clean

We don't need chemical warfare to keep our homes safe.

Real clean smells like nothing. Or like vinegar. Or sunshine. Or the faint sweetness of lemon peel and warm wood.

Simple, Powerful Alternatives:

- White vinegar: Kills bacteria, cuts grease, removes soap scum.

- Baking soda: Gently scrubs, deodorizes, and lifts stains.

- Castile soap: A plant-based, non-toxic multi-purpose cleanser.

- Essential oils (optional): Add antimicrobial properties without synthetic fragrance.

If you prefer store-bought products, look for brands that:

- Fully disclose all ingredients

- Are EWG Verified or MADE SAFE certified

- Avoid quats, phthalates, dyes, and synthetic fragrance

Quick Detox Wins: 5 High-Impact Swaps

1. Ditch disinfectant wipes – Replace with a vinegar + essential oil spray.

2. Switch to unscented laundry detergent – Fragrance-free reduces VOC load dramatically.

3. Replace air fresheners with fresh air – Open a window or simmer herbs on the stove.

4. Use castile soap for floors and counters – Gentle, effective, and safe for all ages.

5. Toss antibacterial everything – Your microbiome will thank you.

The Clean That Heals

This isn't about doing less. It's about doing better.

It's about remembering that you are not just cleaning a house, you are tending to a living space, a space where lungs breathe, skin absorbs, and children grow.

Clean can still mean orderly, safe, and beautiful.

But let it also mean free from poison.
Free from fear.
And full of truth.

Chapter 3:

Microplastic Nation

You can't see them. You can't smell them. But you're likely breathing them, eating them, and wearing them, right now. Microplastics have become one of the most insidious contaminants in our environment, and they've infiltrated every part of the modern home. From laundry lint to tap water, baby bottles to vacuumed dust, these microscopic plastic particles are not just everywhere around us, they're inside us.

A 2022 study published in *Environmental International* found microplastics in 100% of human placentas tested (Ragusa et al., 2022). Another found plastic particles in human blood for the first time, suggesting that microplastics can pass through biological barriers and circulate within the body (Leslie et al., 2022).

We've become a plasticized population, and our homes are ground zero.

Where Microplastics Come From

Microplastics are not just the result of discarded water bottles or ocean pollution. They are woven into the fabric of modern life, literally and figuratively. And most people have no idea how deeply they've infiltrated our homes, bodies, and daily routines.

By definition, microplastics are tiny plastic particles less than 5 millimeters in diameter. They come from two main sources:

1. Primary microplastics: manufactured small particles used in industrial processes or products, like microbeads in face scrubs (now banned in many places).

2. Secondary microplastics: fragments that break off from larger plastic products as they degrade: clothing, packaging, furniture, carpets, even paint.

And these fragments don't just end up in the ocean. They end up in your washing machine. In your air. In your dust. In your food. In your child's mouth.

Clothing and Textiles: The Invisible Shedders

Every time you wash synthetic fabrics—like polyester, fleece, spandex, or nylon—tiny plastic fibers shed into the water. A single load of laundry can release hundreds of thousands of microfibers into the environment. These fibers are too small to be caught by most municipal wastewater systems and end up in rivers, oceans, and soil.

But they don't just escape in water. They also enter the air. Synthetic textiles release fibers as they're worn, moved, or dried. These fibers float invisibly through our homes, landing on food, bedding, toys, and the floor where children crawl.

Soft, cozy pajamas. Plush stuffed animals. Fleece baby blankets. If they're made from synthetic materials, they're shedding microplastics into the environment with every touch.

Plastics in the Kitchen: Heat, Food, and Leaching

Plastic food storage containers, utensils, packaging, and cookware all contribute to microplastic exposure, especially when exposed to heat, friction, or acidic foods.

- Microwaving food in plastic accelerates breakdown.

- Scraping food with plastic utensils causes wear.

- Plastic water bottles left in hot cars or reused over time can shed microfragments.

- Packaged food—especially fatty or salty foods—can leach chemicals from the container into the food itself.

And once they enter the food supply, these plastics don't leave. They move from the stomach to the bloodstream, where they've been detected in human organs, breast milk, and placental tissue.

Household Items That Constantly Shed Microplastics

- Carpets made from polypropylene or nylon

- Upholstered furniture with synthetic covers or foam

- Paints and coatings that contain plastic polymers

- Cleaning sponges and scrubbers made of plastic mesh

- Plastic toys, teethers, and pacifiers

Each of these releases tiny plastic fragments with daily use, friction, wear, or exposure to heat and sunlight. And over time, those fragments accumulate in household dust, where they are ingested, inhaled, and absorbed.

Why This Matters More for Children

Children are especially vulnerable. They play closer to the ground, put objects in their mouths, and have faster metabolisms and immature detox systems. They also breathe more rapidly than adults and are more likely to ingest dust through hand-to-mouth behavior.

In one study, researchers found that infants may ingest 10 to 20 times more microplastics per day than adults, simply because of how much they interact with synthetic materials and indoor dust.

The soft plastic toys we buy to comfort them...
The foam play mats we use to protect them...
The fleece pajamas we put them to bed in...
These may be contributing to the very discomforts and
immune issues we later struggle to explain.

How They Get Into Our Bodies

We ingest microplastics primarily through food, water,
and air. Studies have found microplastics in:

- Bottled water and tap water

- Table salt

- Seafood and produce

- Breastmilk (Valerio et al., 2023)

- Household dust, which is inhaled or ingested
  (especially by children who play close to the floor)

Plastic particles can lodge in tissues, cross the gut
barrier, and carry toxic additives such as BPA, flame
retardants, and heavy metals. The long-term health
consequences are still being studied, but researchers are
concerned about inflammation, immune dysregulation,
hormone disruption, and even reproductive toxicity.

Children and Babies: The Most Exposed

Infants are especially vulnerable. A 2020 study found that babies fed from plastic baby bottles ingest millions of microplastic particles per day (Li et al., 2020). And because babies crawl, mouth toys, and spend more time close to the floor, they're exposed to far more dust-borne microplastics than adults.

The cumulative effect of daily exposure, starting in utero and continuing through early childhood, is profound. Plastic isn't just polluting the planet, it's rewiring our bodies.

What Microplastics Do Inside Us

We used to believe microplastics passed harmlessly through the body. That they were too large to absorb, too inert to matter. But emerging research tells a different story.

Microplastics are not just environmental pollutants. They are biologically active particles that can penetrate tissues, disrupt immune responses, and act as Trojan horses for even more dangerous substances.

They have been detected in:

- Human blood

- Breast milk

- Placental tissue

- Lungs

- Liver and kidney samples

And their size is not a limit, it's a liability. The smaller the particle, the deeper it can go.

From Gut to Bloodstream

When ingested, microplastics travel through the digestive system, and many pass into the bloodstream through tiny gaps in the gut lining. This is especially problematic for people with gut inflammation, leaky gut, or compromised microbiomes, which includes many children, postpartum women, and those with autoimmune conditions.

Once inside the bloodstream, these plastic particles can lodge in organs, irritate tissues, and trigger low-grade inflammation, a root contributor to many chronic diseases.

Endocrine Disruption

Many microplastics are made from polymers like polyethylene, polypropylene, polystyrene, and PET, which often contain additives such as phthalates, bisphenols, flame retardants, and heavy metals. These additives do not stay locked inside the plastic. They leach out slowly over time, and once inside the body, they can mimic or block natural hormones.

This contributes to a wide range of problems:

- Irregular menstrual cycles

- Low testosterone

- Early puberty

- Thyroid dysfunction

- Infertility

- Metabolic imbalance

- Hormonal weight gain

And because these particles are lipophilic—meaning they are fat-loving—they tend to accumulate in fatty tissues, including breast tissue, brain tissue, and the adrenal glands.

Immune System Interference

Microplastics don't just sit there. They confuse and exhaust the immune system. The body recognizes them as foreign invaders but doesn't know how to eliminate them effectively.

This can result in:

- Chronic low-level inflammation

- Immune hypersensitivity

- Exacerbation of allergies and autoimmune conditions

- Slower healing and increased susceptibility to infections

Studies in animal models have shown that microplastic exposure can alter gut bacteria, reduce white blood cell counts, and increase oxidative stress. In humans, researchers are just beginning to understand the long-term effects, but the early signals are deeply concerning.

What We Don't Know (Yet)

We are only beginning to map the ways microplastics move through and affect the human body. Most regulatory agencies are decades behind the science. There are no federal limits for microplastics in food, water, or indoor air. No warnings on fleece pajamas or plastic food containers. No labels telling parents what their babies are chewing on.

And yet the evidence is growing.

Not just in petri dishes and lab rats.
But in real people. In real homes. In mothers. In children. In the nest.

What You Can Do

You can't eliminate all plastic exposure, but you can dramatically reduce it inside your home:

- Choose natural fibers: Wool, cotton, linen, hemp, and silk for clothing, bedding, and rugs.

- Use a microfiber filter: Devices like the Guppyfriend or washing machine filters capture synthetic fibers before they enter water systems.

- Vacuum with HEPA filters: This helps trap plastic-laden dust.

- Avoid plastic in baby products: Opt for glass bottles, wood toys, and organic textiles.

- Minimize plastic containers: Especially for food and drink—heat and wear increase shedding.

Every reduction matters. What you breathe, wear, and touch is shaping your biology in ways we are only beginning to understand.

Up next: Poisoned at Rest - Mattresses, Sofas, and the Flame Retardant Lie

Chapter 4:

Poisoned at Rest

You may not think twice about where you sleep. After all, the bed is the place we associate with restoration, rest, and safety. But what if the very surfaces we lie on for a third of our lives are leaching toxins into our bodies night after night?

Flame retardants, often embedded in mattresses, sofas, pillows, and baby sleep products, were introduced in the name of safety. But mounting research suggests that these chemicals are doing far more harm than good, especially to developing bodies.

The History of a Bad Idea

Plastic was not always a villain.

In its early days, it was hailed as a miracle. Lightweight, flexible, durable, and cheap to produce: plastic changed everything. It was invented to solve problems, not create them.

In the mid-1800s, a material called celluloid was developed as a replacement for ivory. It was used to make billiard balls, combs, and buttons without slaughtering elephants. It was followed by Bakelite in the early 1900s, the first truly synthetic plastic, used in electrical insulators and radios.

Plastics were celebrated as *modern, humane,* even *futuristic.* They would free us from dependence on scarce natural resources. They would make things cleaner, safer, more accessible. By the 1950s, plastic was marketed as a symbol of prosperity. It was colorful, affordable, and exciting.

And then came the tidal wave.

Postwar Plastic Boom

After World War II, petrochemical companies, flush with wartime infrastructure and synthetic chemistry breakthroughs, pivoted to the consumer market. They flooded households with new forms of plastic: polyethylene, polypropylene, polystyrene, PVC. Tupperware. Packaging. Toys. Bottles. Wrappers. Bags. Furniture. Flooring.

By the 1970s, plastic had replaced glass, wood, wool, and cotton in nearly every corner of daily life. It was cheap, disposable, and convenient. No more dishwashing. No more cloth diapers. No more waiting for linens to dry.

But somewhere along the way, convenience became pathology.

Plastic was no longer a smart substitute. It became the default. It became the substance of the system itself. And no one asked what happened when it broke down. Or where it would go. Or what it would do inside the body.

Because plastic doesn't biodegrade. It fragments. It migrates. It enters ecosystems, food chains, oceans, and uteruses. And still we keep producing more.

The Feminization of Plastic

Plastic has always been marketed to women.

It showed up in beauty products, kitchen goods, baby bottles, toys, convenience foods. Ads promised more time, less mess, greater ease. They sold plastic as a form of *liberation.*

But what they were really selling was dependence.
On synthetic packaging.
On processed baby formula.
On "feminine hygiene" products soaked in phthalates.
On cleaning tools that shed into the air and onto our skin.

The burden fell hardest on mothers who were expected to manage homes full of toxic materials without ever being told the truth about what those materials contained. And even now, it's women who buy the plastic toys, wash the plastic bottles, sleep in the synthetic sheets, and field the chronic symptoms that no one can trace.

Plastic as a Design Flaw

From a materials science standpoint, plastic is brilliant. It is strong, stable, and easy to mold. But from a biological standpoint, plastic is a mistake.

It is out of sync with natural cycles.
It resists decomposition.

It leaches chemicals that were never meant to circulate inside living cells.

And worst of all, we designed it to be disposable, even though it lasts for hundreds, even thousands of years.

We built a world on single-use plastic, and then we let it leak into every corner of that world—the oceans, the soil, the bloodstreams of babies not yet born.

This was not just an accident. It was a design flaw that was scaled, normalized, and monetized. And now we are living with the consequences.

Why the Truth Took So Long

The plastic industry, like tobacco and oil before it, spent decades funding disinformation campaigns. They funded research to "prove" plastic's safety. They downplayed harm. They shifted blame onto consumers with anti-litter campaigns and recycling symbols that meant almost nothing.

They convinced an entire generation that plastic pollution was the fault of lazy people who didn't sort their trash, not the result of an unregulated, petrochemical-based economic system. And even now, most government safety regulations around plastics ignore cumulative exposure, microplastic ingestion, and endocrine disruption. There is no required testing for how plastics affect human fertility, neurodevelopment, or the immune system long term.

The burden has fallen on researchers, parents, citizen scientists, and mothers to raise the alarm.

We Know Better Now

We know plastics don't stay in the ocean. They blow into our fields, seep into our water, and shed into our air.
We know plastics don't stay out of the body. They migrate. They cross the placenta. They enter cells.
We know they are not inert. They carry chemicals that affect mood, memory, hormones, digestion, and development.

And now, knowing this, we can ask different questions.
We can make different choices.
We can begin to de-normalize what was never natural to begin with.

Because if plastic was a mistake, it's one we're still allowed to correct.

How Flame Retardants Enter the Body

Flame retardants sound like a safety feature. They were introduced with the promise of protecting lives, especially children, by slowing the spread of fire in furniture, mattresses, pajamas, electronics, and building materials. The name itself makes them sound essential.

But what most people don't realize is that these chemicals are not chemically bonded to the materials they're applied to. They are designed to slowly leach, flake, or shed into the environment. And from there, they find their way into our bodies.

Household Dust: The Primary Exposure Pathway

Over time, flame retardants migrate out of furniture foam, upholstery, mattress covers, curtains, rugs, electronics, and baby gear. They settle into household dust, which becomes a key vehicle for exposure, especially for children.

Dust collects in carpet fibers, toy bins, air vents, and the corners where little ones crawl, snack, and nap. Toddlers are at particularly high risk because:

- They play on the floor

- They frequently put hands and objects in their mouths

- They have smaller bodies, faster metabolisms, and immature detox systems

Studies have shown that children have significantly higher levels of flame retardant compounds like PBDEs in their blood compared to adults living in the same household. This is not theoretical. This is measurable, biological evidence of absorption (*Stapleton et al.*, 2012).

Inhalation and Ingestion

Beyond dust, flame retardants also off-gas into the air, especially in warm rooms or during sleep, when body heat warms the mattress or sofa. These particles bind to airborne dust, which is then:

- Inhaled through the nose and lungs

- Swallowed through hand-to-mouth behavior or contaminated food

- Absorbed through skin contact with treated surfaces

This constant, low-level exposure adds up, especially in a home filled with flame-retardant-treated items.

Breast Milk, Cord Blood, and the Womb

What's even more alarming is how deeply these chemicals penetrate. PBDEs and other flame retardants are lipophilic, meaning they concentrate in fatty tissues. That includes breast tissue and breast milk.

Multiple studies have found flame retardants present in the breast milk of American women at some of the highest levels in the world, especially in homes with older furniture or carpet padding. They have also been detected in:

- Cord blood

- Placental tissue

- Fetal circulation

This means babies are being exposed to flame retardants before they ever touch a mattress, simply by developing in a mother's body burdened by environmental load.

How They Stick Around

Flame retardants like PBDEs are classified as persistent organic pollutants (POPs). They resist breakdown, bioaccumulate in the body, and remain in the environment for years, sometimes decades. Even when banned, they continue to circulate through:

- Hand-me-down furniture

- Used mattresses and car seats

- Thrifted couches and recliners

- Dust carried from one home to another

This persistence means that detox is not just a single act, it is an ongoing, intentional, generational effort.

Who Bears the Burden

The burden is not shared equally. Lower-income families, renters, and communities of color are more likely to live in homes with older, lower-quality furnishings that contain flame retardants. They are more likely to buy secondhand gear without access to clean-label alternatives.

And still, parents are blamed when their child struggles with asthma, attention, or mood issues—without ever being told that the "safety" foam under their child's mattress may be interfering with their development.

This is not personal failure. This is systemic environmental exposure with generational reach.

Who's Most at Risk?

- Infants and toddlers, who sleep up to 16 hours a day and spend more time close to the floor

- Pregnant women, who can pass these chemicals through the placenta

- People with autoimmune, neurological, or endocrine disorders, whose systems are already burdened

A 2017 study from Duke University found that children living in homes with flame-retardant-laden furniture had five times more PBDEs in their blood than those in low-tox homes (Butt et al., 2017).

Greenwashing and the Mattress Industry

The mattress industry is one of the most aggressively greenwashed sectors in the consumer marketplace. And for good reason: parents are paying attention. People are waking up, literally and figuratively, to what they're sleeping on. They're asking about flame retardants, VOCs, and off-gassing. And companies have responded—not always with transparency, but with marketing spin.

Every year, dozens of mattress brands launch with soothing names, botanical fonts, and "clean sleep" promises. They use phrases like:

- "Eco foam"

- "Plant-based blend"

- "Organic cover"

- "Natural comfort layers"

- "Greenguard Gold Certified"

But look closer, and you'll often find the same toxic core materials: polyurethane foam, synthetic latex, polyester quilting, and chemical adhesives. The cover may be organic cotton, but underneath is a soup of petrochemical foam and glued layers, often infused with chemical flame retardants unless otherwise stated.

This is greenwashing in its purest form; using earthy branding and vague language to give the illusion of safety while delivering the same old toxic load.

Certifications That Don't Mean What You Think

Many mattress companies cite certifications that sound reassuring but mean very little in terms of real health protection.

- CertiPUR-US®: Common in "non-toxic" mattresses, this certifies that the polyurethane foam meets *minimal* standards for VOC emissions and certain banned flame retardants. It does not mean the mattress is safe or chemical-free—it just means it meets current (outdated) standards.

- Greenguard Gold: This is a more stringent certification for low VOC emissions, but it does not restrict the use of all harmful flame retardants or plasticizers.

- OEKO-TEX®: This focuses on textiles, not foam or adhesives. A mattress with OEKO-TEX certified fabric can still contain toxic components inside.

None of these certifications guarantee a truly clean sleep surface. But they are heavily used in marketing to build trust with health-conscious families, especially new parents shopping for crib mattresses.

The Natural Latex Illusion

"Natural latex" is another favorite marketing term, but it's often a blend of natural rubber and synthetic latex, which is derived from petroleum. If a mattress does not say 100% natural latex, it likely contains synthetic fillers. And even mattresses made from real latex can still be glued together with formaldehyde-based adhesives or wrapped in non-organic fabric sprayed with flame retardants.

A latex mattress can feel better than memory foam. But "natural" doesn't always mean non-toxic.

How to Spot the Greenwashing

When buying a mattress, especially for a crib or child's bed, ignore the branding and start with what's inside. Ask:

- What materials are used in the core and comfort layers?

- Is it made with polyurethane foam or memory foam?

- What adhesives are used to hold the layers together?

- Is it free from all flame retardants, or just some?

- Is the cotton certified organic?

- Is the wool untreated and used as a natural fire barrier?

If a company avoids these questions, or can't answer them with specificity, you're not buying transparency. You're buying aesthetic reassurance.

The Wellness Aesthetic Is Not a Safety Guarantee

A beige linen cover and a eucalyptus-scented showroom don't make a product non-toxic.
An Instagram ad with a slow-motion baby bouncing on an

"organic" mattress doesn't mean it's free of VOCs.
A plant-based foam still starts with petroleum.

We have to unhook from the idea that "natural-looking"
equals safe.

Real safety is not a vibe.
It's material truth.

Detoxing the Bedroom

If a brand-new mattress isn't in the budget, start with
small changes:

- Add a certified organic wool or cotton mattress
  topper

- Use HEPA vacuuming and frequent dusting to
  reduce airborne toxins

- Place a barrier cover between your body and your
  mattress

- Prioritize detoxing crib mattresses and pillows first

Your bed should be a place of healing, not harm.
And reclaiming that space is one of the most powerful,
personal steps you can take in building a safer home.

Up next: Synthetic Skin - What Our Clothes Are Doing to Our Bodies

Chapter 5:

Synthetic Skin

Clothing touches us more than almost anything else, pressed against our skin, cradling our reproductive organs, wrapped around sleeping children, breathing with us through every hour. And yet, few of us ever stop to ask: *What are these clothes actually made of?* Or more importantly: *What are they doing to us?*

For most of human history, garments were made of natural materials—wool, cotton, flax, hemp, silk—woven slowly, dyed with plants, and worn in communion with the land. Today, more than 60% of all clothing globally is made from synthetic fibers, primarily polyester, nylon, acrylic, and elastane (Textile Exchange, 2022). These are plastic derivatives, petrochemical products made from crude oil and treated with chemical softeners, flame retardants, dyes, and antimicrobials.

And when we wear them, we're not just making a fashion statement. We're participating in an unspoken chemical experiment, one that begins at skin level.

The Hidden Chemistry in Your Closet

Most of us don't think twice about what our clothes are made of. We think about comfort, color, maybe whether something is organic cotton or not. But beyond the label and the feel of the fabric lies a reality that few consumers understand. Modern clothing is soaked, coated, bonded, dyed, and processed with chemicals at nearly every stage of its production.

The average piece of clothing today is not made from natural fibers. It is made from synthetic blends—polyester, nylon, acrylic, rayon, elastane—derived from fossil fuels. These fabrics do not just carry the memory of petroleum; they also carry a complex mix of treatment chemicals, most of which are not disclosed and have never been tested for long-term safety on human skin.

What's in the Fabric?

From the moment raw materials are processed into textiles, chemicals are added to achieve certain characteristics. These can include:

- Formaldehyde-based resins to prevent wrinkles and shrinkage

- Perfluorinated compounds (PFCs) to make clothing water-, oil-, and stain-resistant

- Flame retardants in children's pajamas and uniforms

- Azo dyes, some of which are classified as carcinogenic

- Softening agents and antimicrobials, which can disrupt the skin and gut microbiome

- Optical brighteners and bleach residues used in the finishing stage

These substances are not always fully removed before garments reach consumers. A study published in *Environmental Science & Technology* found that many popular retail garments—including those labeled "organic" or "eco-friendly"—still contained residues of formaldehyde and azo dye byproducts (Luongo et al., 2016).

Even so-called "natural" fabrics like cotton are not exempt. Conventional cotton is one of the most heavily pesticide-treated crops in the world, and cotton textiles are often bleached, dyed, softened, and chemically treated just like synthetics.

How These Chemicals Enter the Body

Skin is not a perfect barrier. It is semi-permeable and highly absorbent, especially in warm, moist areas like underarms, groin, and the backs of knees. Chemicals in clothing can transfer to the skin through sweat, friction, and prolonged contact. This is especially concerning during sleep, when the body is more permeable and detox pathways are active.

Studies have confirmed that certain textile treatments, including flame retardants and phthalates, can migrate from fabric into the skin and bloodstream over time (Saini et al., 2014). Children are again the most vulnerable. Their thinner skin, higher surface area-to-weight ratio, and developing systems make them especially sensitive to contact exposures.

The Problem with "Performance" Fabrics

Many of the most toxic garments are marketed as functional. Moisture-wicking yoga pants, antimicrobial underwear, flame-resistant uniforms, wrinkle-free school shirts. These features may sound helpful, but they often require chemical treatments that contain known endocrine disruptors, neurotoxins, or skin sensitizers.

- Moisture-wicking synthetics often rely on polyester and elastane blends, which shed microplastics and may be treated with triclosan or silver nanoparticles.

- "Odor-resistant" and "anti-microbial" fabrics are often coated with nano-silver or zinc pyrithione, both of which may disrupt skin flora and irritate sensitive tissue.

- Flame-resistant children's sleepwear frequently contains halogenated flame retardants, which have been linked to hormone disruption, thyroid dysfunction, and behavioral issues (Stapleton et al., 2011).

The industry is not required to disclose these treatments unless they make a specific marketing claim. So many of these exposures happen without the consumer's knowledge or consent.

Fast Fashion Means Faster Exposure

In the past, a person might have owned a few garments and worn them often. Today, fast fashion brands encourage constant buying, cheaply made clothes produced in chemically intensive processes. These garments are often not washed before wearing, and some are worn directly on bare skin, particularly by teens and young adults.

Unwashed clothing can carry high levels of chemical residues, including formaldehyde, benzothiazoles, and nonylphenol ethoxylates (NPEs)—all linked to skin irritation and endocrine disruption. A 2020 study found that some fast fashion garments exceeded recommended safety thresholds for skin contact chemicals by over 100-fold (Tang et al., 2020).

Your Closet as a Chemical Reservoir

Over time, your closet becomes a source of indoor chemical pollution. Treated textiles off-gas into bedroom air, and clothing fibers break down into microplastics that settle into household dust. These microfibers are inhaled, ingested, and absorbed, especially by babies and children who play on or near the floor.

We spend nearly a third of our lives in bed, another large portion in close contact with our clothing. And yet most of us give more thought to what we eat than what we wear or sleep on.

But our clothes are in constant contact with our most permeable tissues: the groin, the breasts, the armpits, the belly, the scalp. And for children, their mouths and cheeks and feet.

This contact is not passive. It is chemical exchange.

We Were Never Meant to Wear This Much Plastic

When our ancestors clothed themselves in wool, flax, hemp, or leather, their bodies were wrapped in fibers that breathed and biodegraded. Today, we wear plastic blends that don't break down, don't breathe, and don't belong next to the skin.

The average American wears and sleeps on fabric that may contain:

- Flame retardants

- Petroleum byproducts

- Residual solvents and dyes

- Plastics that break down into microfibers

And the symptoms we blame on "sensitive skin" or "mystery rashes" may, in fact, be the body rejecting what it knows is foreign.

What This Means for the Body

We tend to think of clothing as neutral. As something outside the body. But in reality, what we wear becomes an extension of our internal environment. Our skin is not a wall. It is a living, breathing, semi-permeable organ that plays an active role in detoxification, immune response, and hormonal signaling.

When we wear chemically treated fabrics every day, we are participating in a slow, continuous chemical exchange. The skin absorbs what touches it. The lungs inhale what sheds from it. The microbiome responds to what it's exposed to. And over time, these exposures add up.

Hormonal Disruption

Many textile treatments involve endocrine-disrupting chemicals—substances that mimic or interfere with the body's natural hormones. These include:

- Phthalates used in plastic prints or softeners

- Brominated flame retardants in pajamas and uniforms

- Nonylphenol ethoxylates in detergents and dyes

These compounds have been linked to:

- Irregular menstrual cycles

- Fertility issues

- Low testosterone

- Thyroid disruption

- Early puberty in girls

- Delayed development in boys

The endocrine system is sensitive and deeply interwoven. Even small disruptions, especially over long periods of time, can affect metabolism, mood, reproductive health, and immune regulation.

Skin Sensitivities and Allergies

Many people experience unexplained rashes, itching, eczema, or "mystery hives" that don't respond to typical dermatology treatments. Often, the cause is contact dermatitis or chemical sensitivity triggered by fabric finishes or detergent residues.

Some of the most common culprits include:

- Formaldehyde resins in "wrinkle-free" shirts and sheets

- Azo dyes in bright-colored or black garments

- Fragrance residues from detergent or dryer sheets

- Flame retardants in children's sleepwear

These reactions may not appear immediately. They can build gradually, worsen over time, and spread to areas of the body not directly exposed to the offending fabric.

Disrupted Microbiome and Immune Function

Your skin hosts trillions of microorganisms that form its protective microbiome. These beneficial bacteria help regulate inflammation, defend against pathogens, and communicate with the immune system. When we wear antimicrobial fabrics or treat clothing with synthetic detergents and chemical softeners, we disrupt that ecosystem.

A disrupted skin microbiome can lead to:

- Increased infections

- Chronic inflammation

- Delayed wound healing

- More reactive skin

- Overactivation of the immune system

The gut and skin microbiomes are connected. When one is off-balance, the other often suffers. This may help explain the rise in eczema, psoriasis, and autoimmune skin conditions in children and adults alike.

Bioaccumulation: The Long Game

Even if you don't react right away, your body may still be absorbing and storing these compounds in fat, breast tissue, and organs. Chemicals like flame retardants and plasticizers are lipophilic—they love fat—and they don't leave easily.

They build.
They cross the placenta.
They pass through breast milk.
They become part of a generational story written in blood, not marketing copy.

The symptoms may show up as:

- Brain fog

- Sleep disturbances

- Fertility struggles

- Mood swings

- Weight fluctuations

- Autoimmune flare-ups

And because these symptoms are vague, many women are dismissed, medicated, or gaslit while their environments are never investigated.

You're Not Overreacting. Your Body Is Responding.

If you feel uncomfortable in synthetic clothing, if your baby gets rashes from certain pajamas, if your body relaxes only when wearing natural fibers—that is not hypersensitivity. That is wisdom.

Your body is not trying to inconvenience you. It is alerting you to something that doesn't belong. And the more we listen to those signals, the more power we reclaim.

Because the root of health is not in a supplement or a protocol. It starts with what touches your skin, what fills your air, what lines your home.

And that includes what's in your closet.

The Microplastic Shedding Problem

Synthetic clothing doesn't just expose the skin—it contaminates the entire indoor environment. Every time you wear or wash polyester, it sheds tiny plastic fibers. These microplastics float in the air, settle in dust, and end up in household surfaces and our lungs.

In fact, indoor environments are one of the primary sources of human microplastic exposure (Cox et al., 2019). If you live in a modern home with synthetic carpets, polyester curtains, and a closet full of fast fashion, you're essentially living in a snow globe of invisible plastic fibers.

A Familiar Story

After switching to cloth diapers and organic baby food, one mother, let's call her Renee, still couldn't figure out why her toddler's eczema flared at night. It wasn't until she replaced his polyester fleece pajamas and sheets with organic cotton that the rashes began to fade.

We're told clothing is safe. But safety is rarely tested. Comfort is assumed. But what feels soft on the outside may be silently irritating on the cellular level.

So What Can We Do?

You don't need to throw out your entire wardrobe or spin your own flax (unless you want to!). But there are powerful shifts you can make:

- Prioritize natural fibers: cotton, wool, linen, silk, hemp.

- Start with the items closest to the skin: underwear, pajamas, baby clothes.

- Wash synthetics in a microplastic-catching laundry bag, like Guppyfriend.

- Air out new clothes, or wash them with baking soda and vinegar before wear.

- Say no to "performance wear" with anti-odor or wrinkle-free labels.

Most importantly, *don't trade in self-judgment for green purity.* This is about awareness, not perfection. Even one shift—toward skin-friendly, natural clothing—can dramatically reduce your toxic load.

Chapter 6:

Hormones on the Front Line

Hormones are the silent messengers of the body. They regulate everything from sleep and energy to fertility, mood, metabolism, and immune function. They are precise, intricate, and incredibly sensitive to change. And in our modern homes, they are under near-constant assault.

From the moment we wake up and wash our faces with fragranced cleansers, to the moment we crawl into bed on flame-retardant-treated sheets, we are surrounded by chemicals that interfere with the endocrine system. These are called endocrine-disrupting chemicals (EDCs)—and they are everywhere.

What Are Endocrine Disruptors?

You've probably seen the term before.
Endocrine disruptors.
It sounds technical, vague, maybe a little overblown.

But what it really means is this: something outside the body that hijacks your hormones.

Endocrine disruptors are chemicals that mimic, block, or interfere with the body's natural hormone signals. They can alter how hormones are made, how they travel, where they go, and how cells respond to them. Some overstimulate receptors. Others shut them down. Some confuse your tissues into thinking they've received a signal that never came.

Hormones are not minor players. They regulate everything, from metabolism and sleep to ovulation, mood, memory, libido, blood sugar, immune function, and fetal development.

So when something disrupts that system, the effects are wide-ranging, often delayed, and difficult to trace to a single source. But they are real. They are measurable. And they are happening every day, often in small doses that build up over time.

Where They're Found

Endocrine-disrupting chemicals (EDCs) are not rare. They're everywhere.

Common sources include:

- Phthalates: found in synthetic fragrance, vinyl flooring, shower curtains, and personal care products

- Bisphenols (like BPA and BPS): in plastic containers, receipts, water bottles, and food can linings

- Parabens: in lotions, shampoos, and cosmetics

- Triclosan: in antibacterial soaps and some athletic clothing

- Flame retardants: in mattresses, upholstered furniture, electronics, and sleepwear

- Pesticides and herbicides: on non-organic produce, lawns, and treated wood

- PFAS ("forever chemicals"): in non-stick cookware, stain-resistant fabrics, waterproof gear, and even dental floss

These chemicals do not break down easily. They can remain in the body for years and pass from mother to child during pregnancy and breastfeeding.

How Disruptors Affect the Body

Hormones work in microscopic amounts, picograms, or one trillionth of a gram. That means even tiny exposures to endocrine disruptors can have an outsized effect.

Research has linked EDCs to:

- Irregular periods

- Infertility and miscarriage

- Low sperm count and testosterone

- Thyroid dysfunction

- Polycystic ovary syndrome (PCOS)

- Endometriosis

- Obesity and insulin resistance

- Early puberty in girls

- Delayed development in boys

- Increased risk of breast, prostate, and testicular cancers

For children, EDCs can interfere with normal brain development, stress response, and immune system regulation impacts that may not fully reveal themselves until adolescence or adulthood (Gore et al., 2015).

No Safe Dose?

One of the most alarming things about endocrine disruptors is that they don't follow traditional toxicology models.

With most chemicals, the rule is simple: the dose makes the poison. But with EDCs, even very low doses can have powerful biological effects, particularly during sensitive developmental windows: like gestation, infancy, puberty, or pregnancy.

This is because the endocrine system operates in pulses and feedback loops. A tiny interference at the wrong time can cause a ripple effect that affects hormone balance for years.

And unlike food poisoning or acute allergic reactions, the symptoms of endocrine disruption may be subtle, chronic, or misattributed to other causes, until the pattern becomes too big to ignore.

Why This Matters More for Women and Children

Hormones play an outsized role in female physiology. Ovulation, menstruation, pregnancy, lactation, perimenopause all are hormonally driven processes that rely on delicate chemical signaling. Disrupt those signals, and you disrupt core aspects of health, fertility, mood, metabolism, and memory.

Children are even more sensitive. Their systems are developing. Their hormone receptors are being shaped. And yet, they are being exposed in the womb, in the crib, on the floor, and through breast milk.

The timing of exposure is as critical as the type. And many of these chemicals are still considered "safe" under outdated regulations based on adult male models from decades ago.

You Can't Avoid It All, But You Can Lower the Load

The goal is not to live in fear. It is to live with clarity.

You don't have to eliminate every chemical from your life to make a difference. You just have to reduce the cumulative burden. Small shifts, removing synthetic fragrance, switching to glass food containers, choosing EWG-rated body products, replacing old foam furniture can significantly reduce your daily exposure.

And that shift matters. Especially for the next generation.

Because your hormones were never meant to compete with chemicals. They were meant to respond to your body, your rhythms, your needs, not the marketing trends of the chemical industry.

Symptoms No One Warns You About

You wake up tired, even after a full night's sleep.
You feel bloated, foggy, overstimulated.
Your cycle has shifted, but your labs look "normal."
You used to feel even-keeled. Now you're riding a wave of mood swings and irritability that don't make sense.
Your skin breaks out, your cravings spike, your energy crashes mid-morning, even though you're doing everything "right."

You're not making it up.
And it's not just stress.

These are often the signs of a hormone system under pressure.

But no one tells you this. Instead, you're told to manage your stress.
To sleep more.
To try harder.
To maybe go on the pill, or start an antidepressant, or cut carbs, or "just relax."

Rarely does anyone ask:
What's burdening your system? What's coming into your body, through your skin, air, food, and water, that doesn't belong?

The Invisible Load

Endocrine disruptors don't cause dramatic, overnight symptoms. They whisper. They erode resilience, interrupt rhythm, and dull the feedback loops that keep your hormones humming. The result is a long list of non-specific symptoms that are often normalized or ignored:

- Fatigue that doesn't go away with rest

- Bloating, irregular cycles, or painful periods

- Breast tenderness or fibrocystic changes

- Hair thinning or texture changes

- Anxiety, irritability, or feeling "revved up" inside

- Low libido or vaginal dryness

- Trouble sleeping or waking wired at 3 a.m.

- Skin flare-ups like adult acne, eczema, or rashes

- Cold hands and feet, even in warm weather

- Mood changes that feel hormonal but don't align with your cycle

These symptoms are real biological signals. They're your body trying to adapt to inputs it never evolved to handle.

When the System Is Disrupted

The endocrine system operates in cycles and conversations. When it's disrupted, those cycles become irregular or muted. Cortisol gets louder while progesterone fades. Estrogen becomes dominant or unpredictable. Thyroid hormones slow down. Blood sugar swings get more dramatic.

The body is still trying to function, but it's compensating instead of thriving. And this is where symptoms begin to appear, not as disease, but as imbalance.

The problem is, most traditional healthcare models wait for disease to show up on a test. They are not trained to listen to the body's more subtle cues, especially when coming from women.

Why Women Are So Often Dismissed

There's a long history of women being told their pain is psychological, their fatigue is just "motherhood," their cycle symptoms are normal. But many of these symptoms are early warning signs of hormonal overload, inflammation, or toxic burden.

And because endocrine disruptors don't show up on standard blood panels, most doctors don't test for them. Instead, women are told they're:

- Too sensitive

- Too tired

- Too anxious

- Too emotional

- Too much

But the truth is, we are just more hormonally attuned. Our systems are designed to shift with life—through puberty, pregnancy, breastfeeding, perimenopause. That sensitivity is a strength. And when something is off, we feel it.

Your Body Is Not Broken. It's Communicating.

The next time your cycle shifts, your mood crashes, your skin flares, or your body just feels off, pause.

Ask:

- What have I been exposed to lately?

- What products am I putting on my skin?

- What fabrics am I sleeping in?

- What synthetic scents are in my airspace?

- What's in the food I've been eating or the packaging it came in?

You don't need to obsess. But you do need to observe.
Because your symptoms are not random. They're data.
And your body isn't failing you.
It's alerting you, intelligently, consistently, and wisely.

You don't need to fix yourself.
You need to remove the things that never belonged there in the first place.

Why the Dose Doesn't Make the Poison

Conventional toxicology claims that "the dose makes the poison," meaning small exposures are harmless. But when it comes to hormones, timing and sensitivity matter just as much, if not more, than quantity.

Think of hormones like musical notes in a symphony. It doesn't take a crashing cymbal to ruin the harmony; a single out-of-place flute can throw off the entire piece. EDCs, even in trace amounts, can derail the hormonal balance that keeps us well.

This is especially true for:

- Pregnant women – who may pass these chemicals to developing babies

- Infants and children – whose hormonal systems are still forming

- Teenagers – undergoing rapid hormonal shifts

- Perimenopausal women – whose balance is already in flux

Real Life, Real Impact

Let's take a look at a woman I interviewed, let's call her Amanda. She had been struggling with irregular cycles, heavy periods, brain fog, and sudden weight gain after having her second baby. Doctors ran tests, but everything came back "normal." After stumbling into a rabbit hole of research, she began detoxing her home environment, swapping out scented detergents, tossing the plastic food storage, replacing her mattress, and switching to natural body care.

Within three months, her energy returned. Her cycles began to regulate. She didn't change her diet or exercise. She changed her *environment*—and her hormones responded.

The Hidden Hormone Wreckers in the Home

Every room has its own set of disruptors. Here's what to watch for:

Laundry Room

- Scented detergents → phthalates

- Dryer sheets → synthetic musks

- Fabric softeners → quats (linked to reproductive toxicity)

Bathroom

- Skincare, shampoo, lotion → parabens, phthalates, triclosan

- Feminine hygiene products → pesticide residue, dioxins in conventional cotton

- Air fresheners → synthetic fragrance blend containing endocrine disruptors

Kitchen

- Plastic storage containers → BPA and BPS leaching

- Canned goods → BPA lining

- Nonstick cookware → PFAS ("forever chemicals")

Bedroom

- Flame-retardant-treated mattress and pillows → PBDEs

- Synthetic pajamas and sheets → chemical dyes, formaldehyde

- Dust → accumulates all of the above

Cumulative Exposure Matters

EDCs aren't "one and done" exposures. They accumulate in fat tissues, circulate through breastmilk, and linger in dust. When you layer body wash, perfume, laundry detergent, plastic storage, and a memory foam mattress, you get a cumulative hormonal burden that adds up, day after day.

This is why women often say they feel better after detoxing their homes, even before changing food or supplements. It's not placebo. It's biochemical.

What You Can Do

Rebalancing hormones doesn't always mean prescriptions. Sometimes, it starts at home.

- Switch to fragrance-free or essential oil–based personal care products

- Use glass or stainless steel instead of plastic for food and drink

- Clean with vinegar, baking soda, or trusted low-tox products

- Vacuum with a HEPA filter and dust regularly to reduce chemical load

- Choose organic cotton for underwear, sheets, and pajamas when possible

- Filter your water (especially for PFAS)

And most importantly: don't wait for regulators to catch up. Many EDCs are still legal, still unlabeled, and still marketed to women under the guise of "fresh," "clean," and "safe."

Chapter 7:

The Nervous System in Overdrive

You don't feel like yourself.

You're exhausted, but wired. You forget what you were just saying. You're overwhelmed by the clutter, the noise, the constant sensory assault, and yet, all you did was stay home.

This isn't just burnout. It might be your nervous system reacting to your environment.

Your Brain, On Toxins

Brain fog.
Forgetfulness.
Anxiety for no reason.
Mood swings that seem hormonal, but happen out of sync.
Waking up tired. Feeling overstimulated in normal situations.
Struggling to focus, to follow through, to remember what you were just doing.

These are not signs that you're failing.
They are often signs of a nervous system under chemical stress.

We tend to think of toxins as something that affects the body. But they also affect the brain, and often more subtly, more powerfully, and more persistently than we realize.

The Brain is an Energy-Intensive, Chemically Sensitive Organ

Your brain uses about 20% of your body's total energy. It relies on intricate chemical signaling to regulate everything from focus to memory to mood. It is constantly bathed in neurotransmitters, protected by the blood-brain barrier, and supported by the gut, hormones, and immune system.

But modern environmental toxins—especially those small enough to cross cell membranes or mimic natural chemicals—can interfere with these processes at the most foundational level.

And the result isn't always a seizure or neurological collapse.
It's often a slow erosion of clarity, regulation, and resilience.

Common Neurotoxic Offenders

Certain chemicals are particularly known for their neurotoxic effects, especially in sensitive populations like children, pregnant women, and those with autoimmune or neurological conditions.

These include:

- Phthalates: found in fragrance, plastics, vinyl, and personal care products. Linked to attention issues, hyperactivity, and poor working memory.

- Flame retardants (PBDEs): disrupt thyroid hormone signaling, essential for fetal and early childhood brain development.

- Heavy metals (lead, mercury, aluminum): present in old paint, contaminated water, cookware, and some cosmetics. Known to impair learning, behavior, and emotional regulation.

- Organophosphate pesticides: used on non-organic produce and in some flea and tick treatments. Strongly associated with lower IQ and behavioral disorders in children (Bouchard et al., 2010).

- Formaldehyde and VOCs: off-gassing from furniture, flooring, cleaners, and personal care products. These chemicals can irritate the brain through repeated low-level exposure, leading to headaches, mood swings, and fog.

You're Not Imagining It

If you feel scatterbrained in your own home...
If your anxiety gets worse when you clean with certain sprays...
If your child's mood shifts in certain rooms, or in response to new clothes, furniture, or air fresheners...
There may be more at play than stress or personality. You

may be witnessing the nervous system responding to environmental input.

Research has shown that exposure to synthetic fragrances and VOCs can cause changes in brain wave activity. Animal studies show that even low-level exposure to endocrine disruptors in early life can lead to long-term changes in dopamine, serotonin, and cortisol regulation.

And many of the symptoms—brain fog, overstimulation, low mood, memory lapses—are dismissed in clinical settings as "mom brain" or "normal stress," even when they are clear signs of nervous system overload.

The Body Remembers What the Brain Tries to Normalize

We adapt to dysfunction when it's all we've known. If you've lived in a chemically saturated home, you may not even notice what clean air, clean clothing, and clean touch feel like, until you experience them again.

But your body remembers. And so does your brain.

That sense of calm when you step outside.
The clarity you feel after time in nature.
The way your child suddenly sleeps better after removing a scented detergent.

These are not coincidences. They are physiological recalibrations.

They are your nervous system trying to return to a baseline it hasn't touched in years.

This Is Not About Blame. It's About Resilience

We are not weak because we're sensitive.
We're sensitive because our bodies are intelligent.
And because our environments have changed faster than our biology can adapt.

But when we remove the inputs that confuse, inflame, and dysregulate, something remarkable happens.

The mind clears.
The anxiety lifts.
The noise softens.
The system repairs.

This is not instant. But it is possible.
And it begins with awareness, followed by one clear, sovereign choice at a time.

The Link Between Environment and Emotion

When your home becomes a source of constant chemical input, your vagus nerve—the body's communication superhighway between brain and gut—stays on high alert. Instead of resting and digesting, you're scanning and bracing.

You may feel:

- Restless or agitated in certain rooms

- Overwhelmed by smells you once loved

- Like your mind is "fuzzy" or unreliable

- Emotionally volatile, especially at home

- Panicky without knowing why

This is not weakness. It's wisdom. Your body is telling the truth your culture won't name: *something is wrong in your environment.*

A Familiar Story

When I met Elena, she described herself as a "high-functioning mess." A mother of three, she kept a spotless home, Febreze in every room, plug-ins in the hallway, bleach wipes in the diaper caddy. But she felt awful: constant headaches, extreme fatigue, emotional numbness, and racing thoughts at night.

It wasn't until her youngest started reacting to the scented laundry detergent that she put the pieces together. With each product swap and air purification step, her symptoms began to lift. "It felt like I'd been living in fog, and then someone finally opened a window."

Why Women Are Hit Hardest

Environmental toxins don't affect everyone equally.
They hit women hardest.
Not because we're weaker. But because we are biologically and socially positioned to absorb more, carry more, and clean up more,in every sense of the word.

This isn't just about estrogen. It's about exposure, labor, and legacy.

More Time Indoors, More Contact, More Exposure

Women spend more time indoors, especially during caregiving seasons. We cook, clean, nurse, bathe, and sleep next to children. We wipe down counters, change sheets, spray the air, and scrub the tub. We are more likely to buy the household products, apply the lotions, handle the receipts, and manage the laundry.

And we do most of it on bare skin, with no protection, while inhaling the ambient residue of scented sprays, dryer sheets, cleaning wipes, baby powders, and floor cleaners. Even when we buy "better" products, we're often still steeped in chemicals we were never told to question.

That daily contact translates to chronic exposure. And chronic exposure translates to hormonal confusion, fatigue, inflammation, and a symptom load we're taught to see as normal.

The Hormonal Landscape is More Complex

The female endocrine system is not linear, it's cyclical, dynamic, deeply sensitive to change. We move through phases: follicular, luteal, menstrual, ovulatory. We shift again through pregnancy, postpartum, breastfeeding, perimenopause, and menopause. Each phase is governed by intricate hormonal choreography.

And endocrine disruptors are expert saboteurs.

They mimic estrogen, block progesterone, dysregulate cortisol, confuse thyroid function, and interfere with insulin sensitivity. Even low levels of exposure, especially during vulnerable windows like pregnancy or puberty, can ripple through the entire system causing:

- Irregular cycles

- Infertility or miscarriage

- Mood instability

- PCOS and fibroids

- Thyroid imbalance

- Early menopause

- Brain fog, fatigue, and sleep disruption

The Invisible Labor of Detox

Women are more likely to be the ones researching, buying, swapping, and questioning. We are the ones reading the labels. We're the ones tossing the toxic shampoo, finding the safe mattress, switching to glass containers, ditching the plastic toys. We bear the emotional and logistical weight of cleaning up a mess we didn't create.

And when symptoms still show up—when our kids are itchy, hyper, foggy, or sick—we blame ourselves.
We think we missed something.
We think we're failing.
We carry that too.

But this isn't our failure.
It's the fallout of an industrial system that sold us safety and delivered sickness.

Our Bodies Know Before the Research Catches Up

You don't need a lab test to know your body is reacting.

You don't need a peer-reviewed study to feel the tension, the crash, the inflammation.

You've likely noticed it already:

- The scent that makes your chest tighten

- The detergent that causes a rash

- The couch that triggers headaches

- The shift in your cycle when you're around synthetic fragrance

These aren't sensitivities.
They are responses.
They are wisdom.

This Is Not About Fear—It's About Power

You are not broken.
You are not hysterical.
You are not "too sensitive."

You are part of a long line of women whose bodies have borne the cost of modern convenience.
And now, you're drawing a line.

Because reclaiming your nervous system, your hormones, your clarity—it's not just personal.

It's ancestral. It's maternal. It's political.
It's how the healing begins.

What the Science Shows

Multiple studies have now linked indoor air pollution and synthetic fragrances to neurological symptoms:

- A 2016 study found that fragrance sensitivity affected 34% of Americans, with symptoms including migraines, respiratory distress, and difficulty concentrating (Steinemann, 2016).

- Mold exposure is associated with cognitive dysfunction and memory loss, particularly in vulnerable populations (Miller & Vandenplas, 2011).

- PBDE flame retardants have been shown to impair brain development in children, leading to lower IQ and attention problems (EPA, 2015).

These effects are subtle, cumulative, and often dismissed, but they are very real.

How to Soothe a Triggered System

This isn't about moving into a yurt. It's about reclaiming calm, one layer at a time.

- Ventilate daily. Fresh air is free medicine.

- Clear out synthetic scents. Swap air fresheners, candles, and dryer sheets for essential oils or nothing at all.

- Use a HEPA air purifier in the bedroom or high-use spaces.

- Declutter visual chaos. Mess = sensory noise.

- Ground with natural textures—linen, wool, cotton, wood, stone.

- Practice nervous system hygiene: breathwork, touch, cold water, time outside.

- Pay attention to your body's cues. If you feel anxious in a room—listen.

You're Not Crazy. You're Contaminated.

Let's say that again: you're not crazy.

You're overwhelmed by inputs your ancestors never had to process. Your body is not broken, it's *responsive*. Your nervous system isn't overreacting, it's trying to keep you safe in an environment that is chemically and emotionally chaotic.

And the first step to healing isn't another supplement. It's listening to what your body already knows.

Chapter 8:

The Nursery Trap

The nursery is supposed to be the safest room in the house. It's where we rock, feed, change, and soothe our littlest ones. We wash the sheets in gentle detergent, we choose the "natural" baby wash, and we set up the crib under a mobile of stars and sheep. But what if the very space we've curated with love is also exposing our babies to invisible harm?

The truth is, modern nurseries are chemical minefields. From flame-retardant crib mattresses to plastic toys, synthetic pajamas, and baby wipes soaked in fragrance, our children are born into an environment saturated with chemicals long before they even take their first step.

Small Bodies, Big Exposure

When it comes to environmental toxins, children are not just smaller adults. They are uniquely vulnerable, physically, hormonally, and neurologically. Their bodies are still forming, their detox systems are immature, and their surface area-to-weight ratio makes them more absorbent per pound than any adult.

That means when a baby is exposed to a chemical, they are absorbing more of it, more deeply, for longer, and it's affecting more systems at once.

Why Exposure Hits Harder

Children breathe faster. They drink more water and eat more food per pound of body weight. They absorb more through their skin. Their brains are developing rapidly, and their gut lining, blood-brain barrier, and immune defenses are still under construction.

Every system is wide open.

And when a chemical enters that open system, through skin contact, inhalation, ingestion, or dust, it doesn't just get processed and eliminated like it might in a healthy adult. It can linger. It can interfere. And it can shape how the brain, immune system, and endocrine system develop for life.

What "Low Dose" Really Means for Kids

Many of the products in a typical nursery, like mattresses, changing pads, rugs, and plastic storage bins, release trace amounts of flame retardants, formaldehyde, and phthalates into the air and dust.

Industry will say these amounts are too small to cause harm. But that's based on adult models, not babies. And it ignores the fact that small, repeated doses of hormone-disrupting chemicals can have more impact in a developing child than a large dose would in an adult.

A child's hormonal signals are being written in real time.

And when endocrine disruptors mimic or block those signals, the results can include:

- Delayed or accelerated puberty

- Altered brain development

- Disrupted sleep patterns

- Mood instability

- Greater risk of allergies, asthma, and autoimmune disease later in life

Closer to the Ground, Closer to the Source

Babies spend the majority of their early life close to the floor: crawling, scooting, sleeping on low surfaces, playing on rugs. This puts them in direct contact with the most contaminated layer of indoor air and dust, where heavier chemicals like flame retardants and plasticizers settle.

- Crib mattresses can off-gas directly into their breathing zone.

- Foam-filled baby gear can shed toxic dust into their mouths and hands.

- Clothing treated with stain repellents can transfer chemicals through sweat.

- Plastic toys, teethers, and pacifiers can leach chemicals directly through saliva.

And they aren't just exposed occasionally. They are exposed constantly, with developing bodies that do not yet have the enzymes or detox pathways to filter and eliminate these substances efficiently.

This Is Not About Fragility—It's About Biology

This isn't alarmism. This is how physiology works.

Children are designed to grow in clean environments. They were never meant to be raised in rooms full of endocrine-disrupting dust, off-gassing furniture, and petroleum-based fabrics.
That's not fragility. That's biological common sense.

And this is why so many babies today show signs of discomfort that we've been told are normal:

- Chronic diaper rash

- Eczema by three months

- Trouble sleeping

- Constipation

- Allergic reactions with no clear cause

- Reflux, restlessness, fussiness

Sometimes it's diet.
Sometimes it's gut flora.
But often, it's what surrounds them. What touches their skin. What lines their crib. What floats in the air between the rocker and the rug.

Protecting the Vulnerable Means Changing the Environment

Children can't opt out of exposure. They don't choose their mattresses or pajamas or the materials in their nursery. That's our role. And we are not powerless.

With every product we swap, every window we open, every detergent we ditch, every layer of fragrance we remove, we lift a little more weight off their developing systems.

It doesn't have to be perfect.
But every little reduction matters more when the body is small.
And what we do now—at this early stage—echoes for decades.

Cribs, Mattresses & Flame Retardants

One of the biggest hidden threats is the crib mattress. Most conventional crib mattresses are made with polyurethane foam and treated with flame retardants—chemicals like PBDEs, which have been linked to neurodevelopmental delays, hormone disruption, and reduced IQ in children (EPA, 2015).

Even "waterproof" covers often contain vinyl (PVC), which can off-gas phthalates—another class of endocrine disruptors associated with reproductive and behavioral problems.

Parents are often told these materials are required "for safety." But what's the point of fireproofing a mattress if the child is slowly inhaling or absorbing chemicals linked to cancer and developmental harm?

Baby Wipes, Lotions & Diapers

The average baby goes through 6-10 diaper changes a dayeach one potentially involving products that contain:

- Fragrance (phthalates)

- Parabens (preservatives linked to hormone disruption)

- Phenoxyethanol (linked to skin and eye irritation)

- Propylene glycol (a petroleum-based chemical)

Even "sensitive skin" formulas can include irritants, and the skin on a baby's bottom is thinner and more absorbent than an adult's.

Disposable diapers themselves can contain dioxins (from bleaching processes), synthetic dyes, and superabsorbent polymers that aren't required to be safety tested for long-term exposure.

Clothing & Pajamas

Many baby pajamas, especially those labeled as "flame resistant" are treated with flame-retardant chemicals. These chemicals don't wash out easily, and babies wear them for hours at a time, often while sweating or drooling.

Synthetic fabrics like polyester and fleece also shed microplastics, which are inhaled or ingested during play or sleep. These particles have been detected in human lungs, blood, and even placentas (Leslie et al., 2022).

Natural fibers like cotton or wool can help, but only if they're truly untreated and not coated in chemical softeners or shrink-resistant finishes.

Toys, Bottles, and Teethers

Plastic is everywhere in the nursery. Teething rings, toys, rattles, bottles, pacifiers, play mats, many are made with or coated in materials that release:

- Phthalates (for flexibility)

- BPA or BPS (hormone disruptors in older plastics)

- PVC (which may contain heavy metals and other additives)

Even "BPA-free" products often substitute with BPS, which has similar estrogenic activity.

Some of the most popular toys and baby products are imported with little regulatory oversight, especially those sold through online marketplaces.

A Familiar Story

Jess thought she was doing everything right. She registered for all the organic onesies, bought the "gentle" lavender baby lotion, and scrubbed the nursery floor twice a week. But her baby kept breaking out in rashes, and was colicky every night after sleeping in his crib.

Eventually, she found out the mattress was off-gassing VOCs, and the laundry detergent was packed with synthetic fragrance. Within a week of switching to a breathable, untreated organic mattress and swapping to unscented soap, her baby's skin cleared, and so did her anxiety.

What You Can Do

Rebuilding a safe nursery doesn't mean replacing everything at once. Start small, and focus on what's closest to the baby's skin, lungs, and mouth.

High-impact swaps:

- Crib mattress → untreated organic mattress or natural latex with breathable wool cover

- Baby wipes → water wipes or cloth wipes with warm water

- Laundry detergent → fragrance-free, low-tox options like Branch Basics or Truly Free

- Pajamas → organic cotton or untreated wool, no flame retardants

- Toys & teethers → natural rubber, silicone, or untreated wood

- Air quality → open windows, add a small HEPA purifier, and avoid scented sprays

Bonus tip: Let the baby sleep in your arms more. Your microbiome is safer than the chemical soup we've been sold, and it's great bonding time.

The Nursery Is Not a Showroom

You don't have to build a Pinterest-perfect nursery. You have to build a healing space, a space where your child can grow without silently absorbing poisons wrapped in pastel packaging.

You're not being paranoid. You're being maternal. And the more we speak this truth, the more other mothers will feel permission to listen to their instincts too.

Chapter 9:

From Sickhouse to Sanctuary – Room-by-Room Detox (Without Losing Your Mind)

By now, you've seen the evidence. Our homes, these spaces we've poured our love and energy into are often built from toxic lies. The air, the mattresses, the clothes, the baby wipes... all loaded with chemicals we were never warned about.

It's overwhelming. And for many women, the moment of realization is followed by panic: *I have to fix everything. Right now.*

You don't.

This chapter isn't about ripping your life apart. It's about reclaiming your space in *layers*. Slowly. Thoughtfully. In a way that doesn't burn you out, break your budget, or turn your healing into another performance.

Start Where You Are. Start With What You Use Most.

The truth is, you don't need a 30-step detox plan. You need momentum. You need to start where you are, and take one room, one category, one product at a time.

A simple question to guide the process:

> "What do I (or my child) put on or breathe in every single day?"

Room-by-Room Detox Guide

Bedroom – Start Here. You Spend 1/3 of Your Life Sleeping.

- Ditch synthetic fragrance. That lavender-scented pillow spray? It's usually phthalates in disguise.

- Upgrade your pillow and sheets. Prioritize organic cotton, linen, or wool.

- Vacuum your mattress. Use a HEPA vacuum to reduce dust and flame retardant residue.

- Open your windows. Especially in the morning. Even 10 minutes makes a difference.

- No plug-ins, sprays, or scented candles. They don't belong in your breathing zone.

Kitchen – Where You Store, Heat, and Serve Food

- Replace plastic storage containers with glass or stainless steel. Even BPA-free plastic can leach chemicals.

- Stop microwaving in plastic. Ever.

- Use cast iron, stainless, or ceramic cookware. Nonstick = forever chemicals.

- Filter your water. Especially if you live in an area with PFAS or chlorine contamination.

- Simplify cleaning. White vinegar, baking soda, and unscented soap can replace most sprays.

Bathroom – Where "Self-Care" Often Means Chemical Exposure

- Ditch the synthetic shampoo, lotion, and body wash. Look for EWG-verified or oil-based alternatives.

- Watch out for "natural" greenwashed products. Fragrance-free is better than "coconut vanilla."

- Use less. Seriously. You don't need 9 products to wash your face.

- Replace pads and tampons with organic cotton options. Or try a menstrual cup or disc.

- Toilet cleaner and air freshener? Make your own or go without.

Laundry Room – The Hidden Hormone Disruptor Hotspot

- Fragrance-free detergent is a must. Even "free & clear" often isn't.

- Ditch dryer sheets and fabric softener. Wool dryer balls + a drop of essential oil = done.

- Clean your lint trap and machine regularly. Microplastics and chemical residues build up.

- Consider washing synthetic clothes in a microplastic-catching bag.

Kids' Spaces – Where They Breathe, Crawl, and Explore

- Replace plastic toys with wood, silicone, or fabric. Start with those they mouth or sleep near.

- Open windows and vacuum with a HEPA filter often. Dust is full of toxins.

- Use an air purifier if budget allows. Especially in bedrooms or nurseries.

- Skip the scented baby stuff. They don't need it—and neither do you.

- Don't freak out. Kids are resilient. You're doing more than most by simply being aware.

What Matters Most: Proximity + Frequency + Duration

Don't let Pinterest pressure you into a total aesthetic overhaul. What matters most is *what's closest to your body most often for the longest time.*

That means:

- Pajamas > party dresses

- Crib mattress > nursery paint

- Body lotion > occasional hand soap

- Water filter > organic marble countertops

Focus on daily exposure over one-time events. Prioritize function over form. Remember, you're doing your best, and that is better than anything!

This Is About Power, Not Perfection

There is no such thing as a fully non-toxic life. That's not the goal.

The goal is to create a space that doesn't constantly fight your biology. A space that feels clear, breathable, and real. A space that supports healing, rest, play, and presence.

And that space doesn't have to be magazine-worthy. It has to be yours, truthful, reclaimed, and aligned with what you now know.

Simple Detox Wins to Try This Week

- Open your windows every morning

- Ditch one fragranced product

- Buy one glass jar for leftovers

- Vacuum the mattress

- Swap dryer sheets for wool balls

- Say no to one greenwashed ad

- Take one breath, and remember: you're doing enough

You're Not Behind. You're Ahead

Every time you choose truth over comfort, you're changing the story. You're making space for healing, not just for you, but for your children, your lineage, and everyone who walks into your home.

This isn't about shame. It's about sovereignty. And it starts right where you are, feet on the floor, window cracked, ready to reclaim.

Chapter 10:

The Clean House Myth

We've been taught that a clean house is a moral house. That a clean mother is a good mother. That a spotless kitchen means you're winning at life. But under all that bleach and perfection, something rotten has taken root.

Cleanliness has become a performance. Not a practice of care, but a show of control.

And we've inherited this obsession from a toxic cocktail of patriarchy, white supremacy, class hierarchy, and corporate manipulation. "Clean" isn't just about hygiene anymore, it's a weapon. A social sorting tool. A branding strategy.

And it's hurting us more than it's helping.

How 'Clean' Became a Virtue

Clean hasn't always meant sterile.
Once, clean meant livable.
Fresh air, swept floors, sun-dried linens. A home that smelled like wood smoke and rain. Not lemon-scented disinfectant.

But over the last century, the definition of "clean" has shifted, carefully, strategically, and commercially. It's no longer just about hygiene. It's about morality. Identity. Worth.

Clean became a virtue.
And for women, especially mothers, it became a moral obligation.

From Dust to Deficiency

As consumer products exploded in the 20th century, cleaning was no longer something one did simply to remove dirt—it became a performance of control. Shiny floors, spotless counters, and scent-marked bathrooms became the markers of a "good" woman. A "responsible" mother. A wife who could hold it all together.

This wasn't accidental. It was shaped by advertising, domestic science, and fear-based marketing. Companies told women that cleanliness wasn't just about protecting health, it was about securing love, preserving order, and preventing shame.

Lysol ads once warned wives that neglecting hygiene would lead to divorce. Cleaning brands promised that a well-kept home would protect your children's future, keep your marriage strong, and elevate your place in society.

The subtext was clear:
A messy home meant a messy woman.
And a messy woman was one to blame.

The Smell of Control

Somewhere along the way, we began associating "clean" with scent. Lemon, lavender, pine, fresh linen—chemical illusions of purity, baked into branding. We were trained to believe that if our homes didn't smell like a bottle of something, they weren't truly clean.

But real clean doesn't have a smell.
Real clean is neutral.
Scented products don't prove cleanliness—they cover chemical residue with more chemical residue.

And yet, if a home smells like air or nothing at all, it now feels "off" to many people. That's how deep the conditioning runs.

Cleanliness as a Proxy for Character

For women, especially mothers, cleaning became a proxy for love. We show we care by wiping counters. We prove our value through polished floors and folded laundry. We seek peace in what we can scrub, when the rest of life feels out of control.

But this model of worth is a trap. Because the standard is never satisfied. And the more we try to meet it, while juggling work, motherhood, and our own exhaustion, the more invisible we become under its weight.

What if we stopped measuring our worth in laundry loads?

What if "clean" didn't mean lemon-scented submission, but something far more nourishing?

Why We're So Attached to "Clean"

It's not just about dust. It's not just about germs. Our attachment to "clean" runs deep, because for many of us, clean feels like safety. Like control. Like proof that we are doing okay.

Especially for mothers, the idea of a clean house becomes emotional armor. When everything else feels chaotic—schedules, sleep, school, screen time—we can wipe down the counters. We can control the smell of the bathroom. We can manage the piles, disinfect the toys, fold the towels into some kind of order.

And when that's done, even if nothing else is, we feel like we've held the line.

Clean as a Coping Mechanism

For so many women, "clean" becomes the only tangible thing we can control in a world that asks us to carry too much.

- Clean helps us quiet the internal noise.

- Clean gives us a sense of accomplishment when the deeper work—emotional, relational, generational—feels impossible.

- Clean buys us moments of peace when our nervous system is overstimulated by caregiving, world news, mental load, and hormonal shifts.

But the irony is, the very products we use to create that sense of peace may be stressing our bodies further. The scented sprays. The harsh disinfectants. The synthetic candles and dryer sheets.

They provide a brief emotional lift, but leave a physical burden behind. And over time, our nervous system feels the contradiction.

The Clean House = Good Mother Equation

We've inherited the idea that a clean home means we're doing our job. That visible cleanliness equals love. And that mess, clutter, or grime means failure. Lazy. Disorganized. Undisciplined. Uncaring.

This messaging gets reinforced everywhere, from commercials to Pinterest to pediatric waiting rooms.

A tidy kitchen = nurturing.
Bleached sheets = safety.
No fingerprints on the fridge = you've got it together.

But when this belief goes unchecked, it becomes a self-worth feedback loop:

- If the house is clean, I'm okay.

- If it's not, I'm not.

- If I can't keep up, I must be the problem.

And that pressure doesn't just exhaust us. It prevents us from asking better questions.

The Nervous System Confusion of "Clean"

Your body was never confused. It was conditioned to ignore what it knew.

For generations, women have been told to associate cleanliness with safety. The lemon scent on a freshly wiped counter. The sharp floral cloud of laundry straight from the dryer. The chemical shine of a disinfected bathroom. We learned to interpret these signals as reassurance. If it smells "clean," it must be safe. If the surface sparkles, we can relax. If the air is perfumed, we've done our job.

But the nervous system tells another story.

You may not realize it at first. Maybe it's the subtle tightening of your chest when you use a certain surface spray. The low-level anxiety that seems to settle in after mopping the floor. The headache you brush off as hormonal, even though it always follows your deep-cleaning day. Your body is registering something that your mind has been trained to ignore. And when your nervous system senses chemical chaos—synthetic scents, solvents, VOCs—it responds with confusion, stress, and alertness.

You're not overreacting. You're adapting.

And that's what makes it so hard to spot. Because we adapt to dysfunction. We normalize overstimulation. We tell ourselves it's just stress, just hormones, just the season, just parenthood. But what we rarely consider is that our bodies may be responding appropriately, to an environment that no longer makes sense biologically.

This is the confusion so many women live with: the scent says safe, but the body says no. The bathroom sparkles, but your lungs tighten. The kitchen smells "fresh," but your child's mood shifts. And because we're told that cleanliness equals love, discipline, virtue—we gaslight ourselves. We override the body's quiet intelligence in order to uphold the cultural performance of "clean. But you can't regulate a nervous system in a house full of synthetic signals.

When you begin to detox your home, not just the cabinets, but the meaning of "clean" itself, you may feel more grounded than you've felt in years. You might find that your headaches ease. That your child breathes better. That you sleep more deeply. That your baseline anxiety softens, not because of therapy or supplements, but because your body finally stopped fighting its own environment.

Real clean doesn't smell like chemicals. It doesn't tighten your throat or burn your nose. It smells like nothing. Or maybe it smells like sunlight, and open windows, and sheets dried in fresh air. Real clean is quiet. It doesn't perform.

And when your nervous system stops performing too, you'll remember what safety actually feels like.

Sanitizing the Self

The obsession with "clean" doesn't stop at kitchen counters or disinfected toys. It turns inward. It seeps beneath the skin. And nowhere is that pressure more insidious, or more deeply internalized than in how women are taught to treat their bodies.

From the time we are young, we are taught to believe that our bodies need constant managing. They should be discreet, tidy, and compliant. We learn that to be feminine is to be polished. Smooth. Scented. Controlled. Our bodies are framed not as homes, but as hygiene projects. We are raised to think that the natural functions of our body, sweating, bleeding, growing hair, emitting scent, are signs of something unclean, something shameful.

That belief gets embedded long before we're old enough to question it. And soon we're spending hours and dollars on rituals meant to erase every sign that we are human. Antibacterial wipes. Whitening strips. Vaginal washes. Foaming face cleansers. Bleaching creams. Serums. Toners. Pads designed to block smell, soap designed to foam and "purify," lotions that promise to even and tighten and erase.

What we are sold is cleanliness. What we absorb is shame. And what lingers beneath it all is the idea that we are not acceptable in our natural state.

We've walked this terrain before. In *Skin Deep*, we peeled back the layers of modern beauty culture to expose how fragrance, perfectionism, and shame were sold to women in the name of empowerment, while quietly undermining our hormonal, emotional, and psychological health.

What we're talking about here is the same story, just told through a different lens. The bathroom instead of the vanity. The nursery instead of the makeup bag. The language of purity and safety instead of beauty and glow. But the impact is the same: products that promise power while quietly poisoning the nest.

The deeper tragedy is that many of these products, marketed under the banner of self-care, are quietly compromising the very systems they claim to support. Most are filled with endocrine-disrupting chemicals: phthalates in fragrance, parabens in lotions, triclosan in antibacterial washes, oxybenzone in sunscreens. These chemicals don't just sit on the skin. They absorb. They migrate. They accumulate. And they interfere, especially with estrogen, progesterone, thyroid, cortisol, and testosterone.

We apply these compounds to our breasts, our underarms, our thighs, our faces, the most hormonally sensitive areas of the body. We coat the same tissues that regulate our cycles, support our lymphatic flow, respond to pregnancy, and feed our babies. And we do it because we've been taught that being "clean" means being odorless, poreless, invisible.

But what happens when we internalize that story? When the natural scent of our skin becomes something to erase? When a bit of sweat becomes a source of panic? When softness and stretch marks and underarm hair become problems to fix instead of signs that we are alive?

We start to believe that our bodies are problems. That our biology is a burden. That the evidence of living needs to be scrubbed away.

Even within the "clean beauty" movement, the message often remains the same, just with different packaging. We are still encouraged to refine, polish, correct, and conceal. The goal is still to appear effortless, seamless, pure. It may be safer on the ingredient list, but the deeper pressure hasn't gone anywhere. And it rarely addresses the cumulative exposure of dozens of products layered on daily, or the emotional cost of chasing an unattainable standard.

And this pressure to sanitize doesn't exist in a vacuum. It reflects the larger story: that women must not just be productive and competent, but clean. Not just emotionally steady, but scrubbed of anything too raw or loud or real. Cleanliness becomes a virtue, and the body becomes something to perform, not live in.

But what if we dropped the performance?

What if our skin wasn't a problem?
What if our scent wasn't an apology?
What if the natural texture of our bodies didn't need to be sanded down with chemicals?

What if self-care wasn't about masking, but about listening?

Because the truth is, your body is not dirty. You were never meant to smell like synthetic jasmine or powdered linen. Your womb was not designed to be "freshened." Your thighs were not meant to be reshaped. You were never meant to sterilize your way to worth.

The body is not a project to be sanitized. It is a sovereign, sensing, self-regulating home.
And when we let go of the chemicals, the shame, the messaging, we make space to come back to it.

The Clean = Safe Lie

There's also a deeper lie that needs unpacking: the equation of "clean" with "safe."

We've been sold the idea that dirt = danger. That children must be scrubbed constantly. That a house with fingerprints is a house that failed.

But the truth is:

- A little dirt is microbiome-building.

- A little dust is inevitable.

- A little clutter is a sign of life.

- And real safety doesn't come from sanitization, it comes from connection, awareness, and alignment with nature.

Who Benefits From the Clean House Myth?

If the pressure to keep a perfectly clean, perfectly controlled, perfectly scented home is exhausting, it's worth asking why that pressure exists in the first place. Who does it serve? Who benefits from convincing women that cleanliness is a reflection of their morality, their competence, or their love?

It isn't mothers. It certainly isn't children. It's the corporations selling the problem and the solution in the same breath. The "clean house" myth is not just a social expectation. It is a multibillion-dollar strategy. Behind the pink bottles, floral scents, and feel-good labels are marketing teams, chemical companies, and executives who know exactly how to target maternal instinct and domestic pride. They know that if you can convince a woman her home isn't clean enough, you can sell her more. More detergent. More wipes. More surface sprays, toilet bombs, fragrance plug-ins, hand sanitizers, and bleach-boosted laundry beads. Not because her family is unsafe, but because she might feel like she's failing if she doesn't.

The cleaning aisle is not designed to make your home safer. It is designed to trigger your insecurity, then sell you the illusion of control.

This has been true for generations. In the early 20th century, companies began marketing household products directly to women, using ads that played on fear. Images warned that an unsanitized home would lead to disease, failed marriages, and social embarrassment. Women were told that disinfectant was the modern solution to germs, clutter, and moral decay. After World War II, the chemical industry pivoted from warfare to domesticity, pushing synthetic cleaners, air fresheners, and pesticides into everyday homes. These were sold not only as conveniences but as patriotic symbols of progress. A good mother used modern chemicals. A good wife embraced the future.

Those messages never left. They were just updated with cleaner branding and softer colors.

Today, "clean" is no longer just about sanitation. It is about lifestyle, identity, and performative wellness. Instagram rewards minimalism. Pinterest promotes sparkling white kitchens. And social media algorithms favor fast-cleaning content, quick hacks, and hyper-stylized domestic routines. Behind the scenes, the chemical industry continues to fund "studies" that reinforce the need for disinfection, while lobbying against stricter ingredient disclosure laws. Meanwhile, most cleaning products are still under-regulated. Manufacturers are not required to fully disclose ingredients. The word "fragrance" alone can contain hundreds of undisclosed chemicals, many of which are known hormone disruptors or allergens.

And yet, mothers keep buying. Because we are the ones made to feel responsible for the safety and health of the home. We are the ones told, overtly or subtly, that if our children are sick, our kitchen must not be clean enough. If our partner is irritable, our bathroom must not be fresh enough. If life feels chaotic, we must not be trying hard enough.

But we did not write that script. We inherited it.

And the more we believe it, the more we are separated from our own instincts. We stop asking how our homes actually feel. We stop noticing how certain products affect our breathing, our mood, or our sleep. We dismiss our own discomfort because the label says "safe." We ignore our child's rash because the ad said "gentle." We second-guess ourselves because the messaging is so loud, and our bodies have been taught not to speak.

So who benefits from the myth of the clean house?

The companies that make the sprays.

The brands that scent the air.

The systems that keep women small, busy, and convinced that their worth is tied to how well they manage the mess.

But we don't have to keep playing along.

We can opt out.

We can unlearn.

And we can remember that the people profiting from our exhaustion were never going to hand us peace.

A Familiar Story

Maria spent years keeping her home in immaculate condition. Raised in a culture where "a clean house is a reflection of your soul," she sprayed Lysol daily, wiped her counters with bleach, and loaded up on the "fresh linen" candles everyone raved about.

Then her son developed chronic asthma. Her daughter got recurring rashes. Maria felt like she was always cleaning, but never breathing.

It wasn't until she started reading labels, researching ingredients, and removing scent and chemicals from her home that her children's symptoms improved. And for the first time, she felt like she could *breathe too.*

Reclaiming Clean as Care

Let's take it back. Let's redefine "clean" as:

- The absence of synthetic toxins—not the absence of mess

- The presence of life, not the erasure of it

- The care of the body, not just the illusion of order

- The smell of wood, linen, earth—not manufactured "spring breeze"

Let's choose *ritual over routine, purpose over performance.*

Sweep your floors like a prayer. Make your bed like an act of anchoring. Light a candle for warmth, not for covering shame.

This is not about letting everything go. It's about letting go of the lie that "clean" has to come from a bottle, or at the cost of your health.

Make Room for What Matters

You are allowed to have a house that looks lived in.

You are allowed to leave dishes in the sink.

You are allowed to choose breathability over bleach.

Because your worth has nothing to do with your countertops. And the cleanest thing you can do... might just be throwing out that last toxic spray bottle and breathing deep for the first time.

Chapter 11:

Rewilding the Home

Once we strip the home of toxins, what are we left with?

Air.

Space.

Possibility.

This chapter is about more than what we remove, it's about what we *invite back in*. Because a truly healing home isn't just less toxic, it's more alive.

We're not meant to live in sterile boxes under LED lights, surrounded by plastic and artificial scents. We're meant to live in rhythm with nature, even indoors. Rewilding your home isn't about decorating with driftwood. It's about restoring life to the domestic space.

And it starts with your senses.

Let the Home Breathe Again

A home is a living organism.

But modern construction, synthetic furnishings, and decades of plug-ins and sprays have suffocated that vitality. Rewilding begins by letting air and energy flow again.

- Open the windows. Daily, even in winter. Stale air is toxic air.

- Feel the air move. Use fans and cross-breezes instead of artificial "fresheners."

- Use linen or cotton curtains that move with the wind. Let your home breathe like a body.

The best air purifier? A cracked window and a healthy plant.

Bring in the Wild Textures

Our ancestors lived surrounded by natural materials: wool, clay, wood, stone, straw. These materials regulate humidity, reduce static, and support microbiome diversity. But more than that—they're *grounding*.

What to reintroduce:

- Wool rugs instead of polyester shag

- Linen bedding instead of treated microfiber

- Wooden utensils and bowls

- Stone, terracotta, or unglazed clay objects

- Untreated baskets for storage

These are not aesthetic trends. They're ancestral echoes.

Touch them. Walk barefoot on them. Let your children roll in them. Let your senses come home.

Let There Be (Natural) Light

The nervous system is exquisitely tuned to light cues. But modern lighting, especially LED, fluorescent, and blue screens throws us out of rhythm. It suppresses melatonin, disrupts sleep, and desynchronizes hormones.

Rewilding means restoring the light-dark cycle indoors.

- Open the curtains in the morning. Let sunlight hit your eyes within 30 minutes of waking.

- Use warm, amber lightbulbs instead of harsh white LEDs.

- Dim lights after sunset to mimic dusk.

- Light beeswax or soy candles at night. It's not just ambiance, it's biology.

Bonus tip: Want a happier, more grounded family? Fix the lighting.

Ritual Makes a Space Sacred

We often think of homemaking as drudgery, laundry, crumbs, endless wiping. But in rewilded home culture, every act of care can become ritual.

- Sweeping is a reset.

- Opening windows is a cleansing.

- Folding linens is a meditative act.

- Lighting a candle is a declaration: *This space is held.*

These micro-rituals are ancestral. Universal. And deeply feminine.

You don't need to be spiritual to practice them. You just need to notice what you're doing, and choose to do it with presence.

A Familiar Story

Anika used to hate being home. It felt heavy. Dim. Cluttered. She'd go to Target just to escape, and come home with more plastic she didn't need.

One day, she started small: unplugged the Glade. Opened a window. Swapped her sofa throw for an old wool blanket. Bought a single pothos plant. She noticed the air changed. Then her mood.

Now she lights a beeswax candle every morning while the kettle boils. She sweeps barefoot. Her toddler naps on a floor bed in the sun.

She didn't redecorate. She rewilded.

This Is Your Domain

You don't need to buy your way into a better home. You need to restore your role as keeper of the space. Not in the 1950s "perfect housewife" way, but in the sacred sense.

The hearth is yours.

You are the gatekeeper.

You decide what enters, and what lives here, energetically and physically.

Rewilding is not a return to the past. It's a return to truth. To vitality. To the rhythms we were never meant to forget.

And your home doesn't need to be perfect. It just needs to be *alive*.

Chapter 12:

Bringing the Nest Back to Life

Less About Perfection, More About Permission

Rebuilding your home from the inside out doesn't begin with rules. It begins with *permission* to slow down, to question, to listen, and to change at your own pace. The goal here isn't perfection. It's presence. It's coming back into a relationship with the space that holds you, and the body that moves through it.

You don't need a brand-new house, a spotless pantry, or a perfect toxin-free product lineup. What you need is awareness. What you need is a shift in posture, from obedience to ownership. From performing "clean" to *feeling* well.

The truth is, detoxing the home is not a checklist. It's a conversation with your space. It's the moment you notice that a certain soap gives you a headache, or that your baby sleeps more peacefully after switching out the mattress. It's not about shame or scarcity or panic. It's about remembering that you are allowed to trust yourself. You are allowed to begin exactly where you are.

Your Nervous System Leads the Way

The most powerful detox tool you have isn't a gadget. It's your nervous system.

You've likely felt it already. That tightness in your chest when you walk into a room with plug-in air fresheners. The fog that sets in after cleaning with synthetic sprays. The calm that returns when you open a window or spend the weekend away from home.

These are not mood swings or stress responses. They are data. Your nervous system is designed to sense danger, and not just danger from wild animals or loud noises, but from environmental overwhelm. Synthetic chemicals, chaotic noise, poor lighting, stagnant air, these aren't neutral. They speak to your body. And your body speaks back.

Detoxing the home starts with noticing what brings relief. What helps you breathe. What creates space in your chest and clarity in your mind. This is the wisdom you're rebuilding your life around, not fear, not panic, but regulation.

The Nest Is Still Yours

It's easy to feel betrayed by the home once you realize how many toxins are woven into its fabrics, sprayed into its air, and marketed into its rituals. But the nest is still yours. And it's still worth protecting, not through fear, but through reclamation.

This isn't about throwing everything out or starting over. It's about reclaiming *authority*. It's about saying,

"This space belongs to me. And I get to decide what touches my children, what fills our air, and what rhythms shape our days."

Let the overwhelm pass. You don't have to clean out every drawer overnight. But do let your home start telling you the truth. Pay attention to the items that make you tense, itchy, headachy, irritable. Begin where the resistance is loudest. The rest will follow.

You are not too late. The nest is not too far gone. The body remembers. And when the home begins to heal, the family does too.

You Are Not a Consumer First

One of the most radical realizations you can have in this process is this: *you were never meant to shop your way to safety.* You are not a consumer before you are a mother. You are not a customer before you are a living, sensing human being.

So much of the wellness industry repackages the same toxic narratives under new branding. Clean-label sprays. Organic-looking candles. Subscription detox boxes. And while some of these products can help, they are not where the real change happens.

The shift happens in how you see. In what you question. In what you no longer tolerate. In the moment you realize that the $2 bottle of vinegar cleans just as well as the $12 "natural" disinfectant, and doesn't leave your lungs burning afterward.

You do not have to spend your way to sovereignty. You already have it. And when you act from that place, everything changes.

The Next Generation Is Watching

Your children are not learning from what you say. They're learning from what you live. They're watching how you respond to discomfort, how you navigate change, how you honor your limits and repair what's been harmed.

When they see you replace a scented detergent with something gentle, they learn that safety matters. When they hear you say, "This smell gives me a headache, let's try something else," they learn to trust their bodies. When they watch you open the windows, pause the noise, light a beeswax candle, or step outside barefoot, they learn what regulation looks like in action.

You don't need to be perfect. You just need to be *present*. You just need to show them that change is possible, even when it's slow. That we don't have to live in systems that hurt us. That home can mean something better.

This Is the Work of Repair

There is grief in this process. Grief for what we didn't know. Grief for the exposures we couldn't prevent. Grief for the moments we brushed off discomfort because the label said "safe." But grief isn't the end of the story. It's the beginning of *repair*.

Repair means returning to the body. Repair means questioning inherited habits. Repair means removing what was never meant to be here, and making space for what truly belongs: air, light, quiet, softness, warmth, rhythm.

This work is not glamorous. It doesn't get applause. But it changes everything.

It changes the air your children breathe.
It changes the rhythm your hormones dance to.
It changes how deeply you sleep, how fully you digest, how clearly you think.

This is not a lifestyle trend. This is biological truth. And reclaiming it—one room, one rhythm, one moment at a time—is sacred work.

Be your own hero.

Resources & Citations Appendix

Indoor Air Quality & VOCs

- EPA. (2023). *Indoor Air Quality.* U.S. Environmental
  Protection Agency.
  https://www.epa.gov/indoor-air-quality-iaq
  → Overview of VOCs, mold, ventilation, and
  pollutants in residential buildings.

- California Air Resources Board. (2018). *Consumer
  Products and Air Pollution.*
  https://ww2.arb.ca.gov
  → Found that everyday consumer products emit
  VOCs at levels comparable to automobile pollution.

- NIH. (2021). *Volatile Organic Compounds and Health
  Effects.* National Institutes of Health.
  → Summary of VOC exposure effects on liver,
  kidneys, hormones, and cancer risk.

- WHO. (2009). *Guidelines for Indoor Air Quality:
  Dampness and Mould.* World Health Organization.
  → Found over 30% of homes and buildings show
  signs of mold or moisture-related damage.

Household Cleaning Chemicals

- Environmental Working Group (EWG). (2022). *Hall of Shame: Cleaning Products.*
  https://www.ewg.org
  → Independent review of toxic ingredients in major household cleaners, including "greenwashed" brands.

- Svanes, C., et al. (2018). *Cleaning at Home and at Work in Relation to Lung Function Decline and Airway Obstruction.*
  American Journal of Respiratory and Critical Care Medicine, 197(9).
  → Women who used cleaning products regularly experienced lung decline similar to smoking a pack of cigarettes a day.

Children's Vulnerability & Early Exposure

- Bouchard, M. F., et al. (2010).
  Attention-deficit/hyperactivity disorder and urinary metabolites of organophosphate pesticides.
  Pediatrics, 125(6): e1270–e1277.
  → Found strong correlation between pesticide exposure and behavioral disorders in children.

- Herbstman, J. B., et al. (2010). *Prenatal exposure to PBDEs and neurodevelopment.*
  Environmental Health Perspectives, 118(5): 712–719.
  → Prenatal flame retardant exposure linked to reduced IQ and attention in children.

- Sathyanarayana, S., et al. (2011). *Phthalates and children's health.*
  Pediatrics, 128(5): e1270–e1284.
  → Linked phthalate exposure to abnormal reproductive development and asthma in children.

Furniture, Mattresses & Flame Retardants

- Stapleton, H. M., et al. (2011). *Identification of flame retardants in foam collected from baby products.*
  Environmental Science & Technology, 45(12), 5323–5331.
  → Revealed widespread use of toxic flame retardants in crib mattresses, changing pads, and nursery chairs.

- Luongo, G., et al. (2016). *Chemicals in clothing: Formaldehyde and arylamines in new garments.*
  Environmental Science: Processes & Impacts, 18, 1035–1042.
  → Found formaldehyde in clothing at levels high

enough to cause skin reactions.

Endocrine Disruption & Hormonal Health

- Gore, A. C., et al. (2015). *EDCs and public health: Effects on development and health outcomes.* Endocrine Reviews, 36(6), E1–E150.
  → Comprehensive report on how endocrine disruptors affect fertility, puberty, pregnancy, thyroid, and brain development.

- Rochester, J. R. (2013). *Bisphenol A and human health: A review of the literature.* Reproductive Toxicology, 42, 132–155.
  → Reviewed impacts of BPA on hormone disruption and reproductive health.

- Engel, S. M., et al. (2010). *Prenatal phthalate exposure and behavior in children.* Environmental Health Perspectives, 118(4), 565–571.
  → Associations between maternal phthalate exposure and behavioral issues in children.

Neurotoxins & Mental Health Impact

- Lanphear, B. P., et al. (2005). *Low-level environmental lead exposure and children's intellectual function.*
  Environmental Health Perspectives, 113(7): 894–899.
  → Demonstrated that even very low levels of lead impact cognitive performance in children.

- Leslie, H. A., et al. (2022). *Discovery and quantification of plastic particle pollution in human blood.*
  Environment International, 163, 107199.
  → First study to detect microplastics circulating in human bloodstream.

- Tang, S., et al. (2020). *Hazardous chemicals in fast fashion garments.*
  Journal of Hazardous Materials, 403, 123914.
  → Found over 100x safety limits for skin-contact chemicals in some fast fashion brands.

Pregnancy, Breastmilk & Generational Impact

- Toms, L.-M. L., et al. (2009). *PBDEs in human milk: Temporal trends and infant exposure.*
  Environment International, 35(6), 929–935.
  → Flame retardants detected in breast milk samples; levels higher in households with newer

furnishings.

- Stapleton, H. M., et al. (2012). *Flame retardants in house dust and hormone levels in men and women.* Environmental Health Perspectives, 120(1), 93–98.
  → Found measurable hormone disruption from household dust contaminated by treated furniture.

Tools & Directories for Low-Tox Living

- Environmental Working Group (EWG):
  https://www.ewg.org
  → Skin Deep database, Guide to Healthy Cleaning, tap water testing, and product safety rankings.

- Made Safe Certification:
  https://www.madesafe.org
  → Comprehensive vetting of household and personal care products with strict ingredient screening.

- Think Dirty App:
  https://www.thinkdirtyapp.com
  → Ingredient breakdowns for cosmetics and body care. Helpful for on-the-go shopping.

- EWG Healthy Living App:
  [Available on iOS + Android]

→ Scan barcodes to get toxicity ratings and ingredient alerts for thousands of products.

Recommended Reading

Environmental Health & Toxic Exposure

- Slow Death by Rubber Duck by Rick Smith & Bruce Lourie
  A groundbreaking and accessible look into how everyday products poison us—and what to do about it.

- A Poison Like No Other by Matt Simon
  A sharp, investigative deep dive into microplastics and their infiltration into every corner of modern life.

- Toxic Exposures by Susan L. Smith
  A historical and feminist exploration of environmental toxins, public health, and reproductive consequences.

- The Body Toxic by Nena Baker
  An investigative classic exploring how chemicals enter our bodies and how industry keeps them there.

Home Detox & Maternal Ecology

- Healthy Child, Healthy World by Christopher
  Gavigan
  A clear, gentle guide to reducing environmental
  toxins in the home, especially during pregnancy and
  early childhood.

- Detox Your Home by Christine Dimmick
  Straightforward and action-based, this is a solid
  primer on low-tox home living with practical
  suggestions.

- Beyond Labels by Joel Salatin & Sina McCullough
  A discussion between two generations on
  reclaiming food, medicine, and health from
  industrial systems.

Hormonal & Nervous System Repair

- The Invisible Kingdom by Meghan O'Rourke
  A poetic and personal memoir that maps the
  terrain of chronic illness, medical gaslighting, and
  sovereign healing.

- The Fifth Vital Sign by Lisa Hendrickson-Jack
  A powerful reframing of the menstrual cycle as a vital health marker, and a call for body literacy in women.

- Burnout by Emily & Amelia Nagoski
  A nervous-system-based approach to female overwhelm that pairs beautifully with your home detox journey.

Ancestral, Feminine, & Embodied Wisdom

- Witch: Unleashed. Untamed. Unapologetic. by Lisa Lister
  A fierce reclamation of body wisdom, cycle power, and feminine sovereignty.

- Braiding Sweetgrass by Robin Wall Kimmerer
  A lyrical weaving of Indigenous science, motherhood, ecology, and relational living.

- Women Who Run With the Wolves by Clarissa Pinkola Estés
  An archetypal, deep-medicine exploration of the wild feminine, storytelling, and reclamation.

Made in the USA
Monee, IL
25 May 2025

18147668R00099